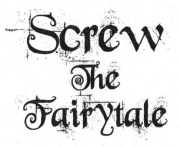

Screw
The
Fairytale

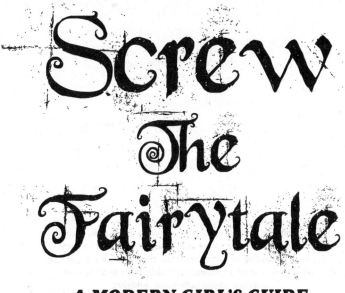

Screw The Fairytale

A MODERN GIRL'S GUIDE TO SEX AND LOVE

Helen Croydon

JOHN BLAKE

Published by John Blake Publishing Ltd,
3 Bramber Court, 2 Bramber Road,
LondonW14 9PB, England

www.johnblakepublishing.co.uk

www.facebook.com/Johnblakepub facebook
twitter.com/johnblakepub twitter

First published in 2014

ISBN: 978-1-78219-750-8

The right of Helen Croydon to be identified as the author of this work has been
asserted by her in accordance with the Copyright, Designs and Patents Act 1988.

Papers used by John Blake Publishing are natural, recyclable products made
from wood grown in sustainable forests. The manufacturing processes
conform to the environmental regulations of the country of origin.

Every attempt has been made to contact the relevant copyright-holders,
but some were unobtainable. We would be grateful if the
appropriate people could contact us.

All facts and figures were correct at the time of publication.

Contents

Acknowledgements

The raw ingredients for this book have been the many people who feature in it. These pages would certainly not exist had I not come across so many willing, open and co-operative interviewees. Thank you to everyone who gave me their time to tell their stories for this book, and to those who didn't know their stories would appear in a book but graciously agreed! I have of course disguised you all and it would ruin it if I named you here, but if you feature beyond this page, thank you.

I am hugely grateful to the organisations and websites who helped me find interviewees and case studies namely, the asexuality support group AVEN, the organisers of Poly Day, Little Sins, which organises swingers parties, the dating websites maritalaffair.co.uk, sugardaddie.com, seekingarrangment.com, anastasiadate.com and the many helpful members of the BDSM community.

I'd also like to thank my wonderful friends, family and acquaintances for their unending supply of anecdotes about their own relationship experiences or opinions (and for pointing me in the direction of others with even more colourful anecdotes). Not everything comes from controlled interview conditions of course and if on any page, you happen to think: 'Oh my god, she's talking about me,' (mainly my married friends or those with kids) then I'm probably not. Or if I am, I exaggerated for the purpose of art. I am a writer. That's what I do! I promise, no negative character judgements about any married friends or mothers of small children have been made in the writing of this book.

I am also indebted to my friend and colleague, the sociologist Catherine Hakim for her diligent fact checking of social science research and other much welcomed feedback. Also, marriage historian Stephanie Coontz for allowing me to reference her work and fact checking a huge chunk of text relating to the history of marriage; Dr Helen Fisher for her help and co-operation with explaining the science of romantic love. Her research into this fascinating concept has been the single biggest revelation for me when it comes to understanding the human condition of love. The work of historian Elizabeth Abbot in *Mistresses: A History of the Other Woman* has also been a huge help to a chunk of this book.

I'd like to thank my agent Andrew Lownie for his unwavering perseverance and keeping up with its many formats as I jumped from a memoir to social commentary to self-help to a memoir again and eventually to journalistic reportage. Also, all the team and editors at John Blake for their help particularly Clare Christian and Rosie Virgo who have been so efficient in coordinating everything.

Finally, thanks to my mum, sister and family for continuing to support my controversial choice of writing topic and for

ACKNOWLEDGEMENTS

not acting shocked whenever revelations from my love life go public (I'm afraid there are a few more confessional parts in this book, but not many!). On the same note, I'd like to thank my friends for cheering on a writer who doesn't always represent the most popular views. Many of you even showed my first book to your mums despite its content! Loyalty doesn't get better than that. Particular thanks to Catherine O for continuing to buy and plug all my work to everyone she ever meets, and to those who have lifted my spirits when I've encountered a nasty online comment or two. A heartfelt thanks goes to Chris Fowler, a special friend and springboard for ideas at the time of writing this book. And a big high five to my appointed humour checker Suki Bains for reading snippets of this book and telling me honestly whether it was funny or not. If it's not, it's all her fault!

Introduction

On life's list of priorities, I'd put marriage and kids somewhere around position 3,996, maybe just before tightrope walking across the Grand Canyon and just after booking to get liposuction in my toes (some women actually do that). It's not that I'd rule any of these things totally out, it's just that none of the above would add to my life in any way and there are more appealing things I'd rather do.

I've never really been the settling down type. My parents didn't divorce or hate each other. An ex never ran off with a best friend (to my knowledge). No one ever left me on the hard shoulder of a motorway after a row; I haven't been bitterly pipped to a job post by a man. I haven't even been dumped that many times! It's just that I feel like I wilt when I'm in a relationship and I've always thrived most when single. I've always felt that my thirst for life, my spark, my energy, my *joi de vivre*, my productivity, my career, my health, my sleep, my gym routine, my friendships, my libido and everything else have been best when there's just me to juggle them all.

Of course there are many wonderful things about being in a full-time relationship and many of them feature in my happiest memories but for all their cosiness they always become overshadowed by sense of duty. I don't feel like I can do all the things I want to do with my time any more. There's less spontaneity about life. I can't choose where I go on holiday; I don't have the right to say I want to stay at home all weekend on my own and read three books in my pyjamas. That vague life plan to one day uproot and move to an exotic climate seems ever fainter.

But I've had fabulous relationships. I've been with men who have adored me, promised me everything and told me they'll never leave. In turn I've loved them as wholeheartedly back but I've often broken their hearts because there always comes a point when I wanted to go back to my roots: to being single. For me, after the initial, wonderful high of romantic love settles, a relationship starts to feel more like an obligation than a desire. I've broken my own heart too because I've walked away from men that I really loved because I wanted my freedom back. No matter how much either half of a couple wants out, it's searing to throw away those months or years of shared history, private jokes and that built-up intimate understanding.

When I started writing this book, I had been single for six years with a series of what I call 'low-maintenance lovers'. Not casual fuck buddies but meaningful connections. 'I don't have boyfriends, I have lovers!' was my mischievous tagline whenever a random stranger probed for my relationship status. A low-maintenance lover offers continuity, regularity and lots of mutual respect and affection but there's no expectation to fit shelves, no anxiety about longevity and no obligation to learn friends' names. I wanted for nothing more. Then halfway through this book, I fell in love. Not one of my usual low-maintenance lovers, whom I saw a couple of times a month, but a proper, committed, invested boyfriend. It was hard to adapt at first after six years of being my own agent. But for all my pro-single life views, it felt wonderful to be in love and to be loved and to feel a secure sense of belonging with someone. I started to believe that maybe I was wrong and the fairytale ending is actually what we all want after all?

But no. I soon felt myself gravitating back to my default setting. My affection and care for the 'proper boyfriend' didn't wane but excitement for the relationship did, as well as my tolerance to operate as a half of a couple instead of as an individual. As devastating and hurtful as it was for me to break away, it confirmed once more that for me, and many people like me, we operate better as independent individuals, our lives punctuated with wonderful and rewarding romances. I call us the serial singletons. We're not anti-love. In fact our romances are our big highs but we live off the buzz of romantic love and when that starts to turn into domesticity and watching TV together, passion turns to routine sex, conversations become shorter and we find our time is being taken up by relationship maintenance, well, we start to feel caged and wonder whether we would thrive better out of it. That may sound like we have no staying power or we lack commitment. But actually, why is that so wrong? In today's increasingly autonomous world it is possible to function brilliantly alone and possible to meet new people at different stages of our lives, so why should we aspire to self-denial?

Popular wisdom has us believe that we will find a

partner who will 'complete' us. For many, I'm sure they do. Some people cannot survive without their rock backstage, guiding them through life's maze of events but for me, I've always felt having a partner always in the shadows takes something away.

For most of us, our views on relationships and building a family are underpinned by what I call the fairytale narrative. We are instilled with the belief that we will all meet a soul mate that understands us and live happily ever after. The only route to Utopia is via a committed, life-long, full-time cohabiting relationship. A relationship's success is judged on its longevity.

People put all sorts of life decisions on hold while they await the arrival of a mysterious stranger. One single friend says she is putting off purchasing her first property, even though she has the means to do so, 'in case she meets someone'. People blame their foibles on not having a partner. One friend is convinced her writer's block is because she doesn't have a boyfriend. Another thinks she'd get fit if she found a boyfriend who was into fitness.

When we do meet someone, we are so obsessed with living out the fairytale narrative that we place huge demands on them to integrate with our lives. We try to change their habits and routine, we disapprove of their friends that we don't like. We claim them as our property, promptly extinguishing all romantic sparks. We spend the first few wonderful weeks gazing at each over a glass of wine, giggling and lying in bed until noon. No sooner has the sore head cleared than we are merging our furniture, pictures, CDs and soon our identities because this is The One. Every week one of my Facebook friends changes their surname and marks themselves as 'married'. I always think it seems like five minutes since I was with that ex-colleague/friend of friend/ acquaintance in a bar while they talked about their hopes and ambitions for life, one that didn't have anything to do with their now-spouse.

Anything that doesn't fit with the fairytale narrative is reproached. As I enjoyed a vibrant life of low-maintenance lovers whom I saw two to three times per month, the only downside was batting off opposition to it. Every day was like fending off a single-lifestyle coup! Well-meaning friends or loved ones took it upon themselves to fix me up. Surely I could not feel complete as a singleton? Of course I'd be happier hitched up with one of their friends or colleagues, or that nice boy we met at the BBQ the week before?

Constant companionship and having someone to build and share a home may well be some people's ideal. But it certainly wouldn't suit me and I'm not alone. Some people, I have noted, are never, ever single. Like temp jobs, I have several friends who hop between relationships. One comes to an end, it's catastrophic, they call in sick for a week and then suddenly two weeks later their Facebook status pops up with 'in a relationship' followed by a picture showing them glued to the cheekbone of their new beau. It gets 57 'likes'. Everyone's relieved, a happy ending – phew! But I can't help thinking, how can they have found genuine love so quickly? Before my 'proper boyfriend', I hadn't met anyone for six years whose vocal chords I hadn't secretly wished would vaporise after spending more than twenty-four hours together. Could it be that many people sub-consciously convince themselves to fall in love because being in a relationship facilitates life in some way?

If I was one of those girls whose goal was to get a ring on my finger, or if I was lonely, bored, or concerned about my declining fertility, then I would have made things work with the proper boyfriend. Or more likely, at the age of 36, I'd already be married.

You might just think I'm cold-hearted so I'm going to go into practical matters. These may sound like small things, but there are two basic reasons that put me off a conventional full-time relationship. First, I absolutely cannot share a bed. 'You'll get used to it,' my married friends assure me as if it's something I must do. I've 'got used' to wet British summers and commuter's armpits being stuffed in my face on the Tube in rush hour, neither of which I have taken a natural taking to. Why would I voluntarily give up my quality REM-ing if I don't need to? And for the record, I lived with one man for two whole years and I *never* got used to it. When he finally moved out, after seven nights of undisturbed sleep, people kept telling me how fresh I looked.

If you're a man, chances are you will think I'm being ridiculous. But I attest, I wake up to the crack of a lover's toe and I won't get back to sleep again! The men with whom I've been on shared-bed terms seem to slip in and out of sleep like it's the Hokey Cokey. Numerous studies show that women sleep more lightly than men and find it harder to get back to sleep once woken. Arianna Huffington of *The Huffington Post* once declared sleep will be 'the next feminist issue'. It's not just being woken while a man is in my bed, it's the waiting for them to get there in the first place! I can recall several times when I've wanted to go to bed before a boyfriend but I've lain there like a lemon, *knowing* I'm about to be disturbed.

Get separate beds, you say. A fair suggestion, but what about holidays or while staying with friends? Should I request a separate room? Actually, I have been known, while on a five-day break with a previous boyfriend, to pay for a separate room on day three just to get some catch-up. I did it all on my own credit card so no sweat for him, but phew the grief! I had to console him for a whole hour. No, nothing is wrong. No, I'm not angry. No, it's nothing to do with an argument we had over map reading this morning. Yes, of course I want to wake up with you but it's 32 degrees even at night, we have no aircon, you snore and I just want to sleep!

God really gave women the raw deal on sleeping. Not only do we wake from our slumber more easily but men tend to snore more. In fact, 60 per cent of men compared to 40 per cent of women over 50. What surprises me is there's no drop-down box on Internet dating profiles to forewarn whether your potential Romeo snorts like a pig after lights-out. We get a heads-up if they are a smoker, 'athletic' or have 'a few extra pounds' and whether they're a 'social drinker' or 'drink heavily'. But we will never know if he's a snorer until we invest in at least a few dates and a sleepover. I'm surprised sleep deprived women are not asking for their money back!

But men aren't even embarrassed by their snoring. If women were the more nasally challenged sex, we'd be so ashamed, we'd have our throat nodules botoxed and inner noses waxed because we're so much more apologetic about our unseemly attributes! Men unashamedly snore away. Some even think it's funny.

Anyway, the second seemingly minor but actually massive relationship turn-off is the tricky business of contraception. I know, I know, it's the twenty-first century and we were supposed to have had that sorted decades ago. But we *so* haven't. If a regular relationship meant I had to go on the contraceptive pill, I'd stay single forever.

I'm no defeatist. Many times I have attempted to ingest these hormones and always I've ended up fat, grumpy, spotty, tired, tearful, cold, with permanent pins and needles in my feet, a daily headache and a sex-drive lobotomy. Most alternatives also involve hormones, which have the same, albeit lesser, effect. That leaves condoms, which have a whole set of politics of their own.

For a man one of the advantages of having a steady girlfriend is that he can very reasonably suggest that they go bareback – something which would likely get a slap and a prompt call to a cab company if he suggested any such thing to a casual lover. Once he has shown some commitment, however, almost certainly he's hoping his girlfriend will sort out some sort of long-term contraception. And he has a point – going condom-free is more fun for everyone. But I think men regard the Pill as a magical panacea to the consequences of sex when in fact it's a personality-changing drug.

In the brief interludes of my serial singledom, when I have been in serious relationships there have been attempts with the coil (*bad* periods), the diaphragm (uncomfortable, fiddly, makes an embarrassing noise and you never know it's in right); also, *au naturale*, which proved most unreliable – the consequences of which were emotional, painful, humiliating and expensive.

I don't have this problem being single with lovers: because lovers don't mind coating their armoury in a veil of latex. Suggest that to a full-time boyfriend and I guarantee there will be a sulk. I'm not saying we should all stay single and have casual sex until some pharmaceutical giant comes up with a hormone-free way to prevent unwanted conception but the challenge of contraception adds to the overall faff of a relationship.

You may not relate to all this relationship bashing. That's understandable. Obviously there has to be something rewarding about coupling up otherwise love would not have been the focus of some of the finest works of literature, theatre and other art forms for thousands of years. Nor would the Internet dating industry be worth £2 billion worldwide according to a widely quoted investigation by *The Huffington Post* in 2012.

I feel it too. Just because there are many things about a relationship that put me off, that doesn't mean that I don't want to fall in love again. There are many days when I crave a special relationship; times when I feel I have so much love inside me, ready to shower on someone. There are many sunny evenings when I'd love to be greeted by a handsome familiar face and share a bottle of something chilled on a riverbank. There are times when I want to share a deep secret with someone I truly trust; times when I'd like someone to give me honest, impartial advice or when I want an arm around me as I fall asleep (so long as he doesn't snore!).

Romantic love is the greatest human high of all; it's exhilarating. I'm not scared of love or too lascivious to promise monogamy. I'm not so possessive of my time that I don't want to spend it doing things for people I love. And it's not that my emotions are as hard as steel and I don't need to sometimes turn to someone else for moral support. What I'm overwhelmingly daunted by is the extortionate price of freedom demanded by the modern model of a committed relationship. Relationships these days have become life mergers. I want to fall in love but must I always go on holiday with him? Must I attend his friends' weddings when I hardly know them and corroborate on every weekend diary entry? When we fall in love, we are expected to put that person before anything or anyone else. It's expected that if you are serious you will one day live together and share *everything*. With such a daunting job description, it's no wonder so many people feel weighed down by the demands of their partners and why others avoid a truly intimate relationship altogether.

I like the idea that there is someone special out there just for me, the prospect that one day I'll meet an intimate, special friend. But it's never quite like that for in reality they simply get in the way. They muck up my flat, they leave me with little time for my friends and they disrupt my sleep. I love the affection and tenderness but it's a bit like having a lovely fluffy cat on your knee – therapeutic for a while but then you want to shake it off and just get on with stuff.

In 2011 the writer Tracy McMillan wrote an article 'Why You're Not Married Yet', which went viral and then became a book. According to McMillan there are eight reasons why women around my age (36) are still single. Among them they're a bitch, they're crazy, they're a slut or they're just plain selfish.

Selfish? Why, because I'm depriving some guy of a girlfriend? It would be selfish if I expected the good stuff from a relationship but I wasn't prepared to invest the time. But you'll never find me moaning that I don't have someone at home to give me a shoulder rub (I have no fewer than five different types of masseuse in my phonebook) or that I don't have anyone to do my DIY. If I got myself a boyfriend for the good stuff but secretly resented all the Saturdays he took up, wouldn't that be more selfish?

As I'll explain in later chapters, for most of history life-long partnerships have never been about magical connections and emotional fulfilment. We didn't put love on such a grand pedestal as we do today. Spouses maintained a healthy distance: they had separate friends, social activities, roles, and they preserved some secrets. Passionate love affairs were usually conducted outside of marriage and weren't expected to last long. The idea that you could share intimacies, joys and sorrows with the same person with whom you share your home, family life, domestic chores, children and inheritance was considered unrealistic, dull or even threatening.

There is much irony in the fact that we now live in an era where we need relationships less, yet more than ever we cling on to the ideal of everlasting love. No one has challenged why long-term relationships are considered to be Nirvana. Is it anthropology – the urge to pair up for life being innate, or perhaps social conditioning, religion, or political conspiracy because coupling suits the order of society?

I feel a little like Columbus when he set out to discover whether the earth really was flat, as everyone thought. I want to look at other models of relationships in our modern world. The fairytale marriage, kids, family days out and a chaotic house surely can't be everyone's ideal? After all, life expectancy is on the increase so 'life-long' is a lot longer than it used to be. Convenience-driven lifestyles have made living alone viable. Social media has expanded our social reach so loneliness is less of a threat. Geographical mobility allows more alternatives to settling down. Modern society encourages individualism and autonomy. These things can only make the nuclear, life-long, family set-up more challenging. What is there for romantics like me, who long for meaningful love but don't want the cohabiting 24-7 clause?

Over a period of two years I tracked down and visited as many people in non-conventional relationships as I could. I talked to and met with committed couples who live apart, those in open relationships, asexual couples, co-parents who've never been lovers at all, dominants and submissives, and people like me who consider singledom a lifestyle choice whether they have children or not. Often it meant me visiting events or networking groups undercover so that I could give an untempered reflection of those driven to use marital affair dating websites or the raw emotion inside a sex and love addiction help group. I wanted to investigate the science of love too. Why does it put us in such a fervent state and why, despite the evidence of multiple sexual partners in every single culture in every single era, does society still insist that lifelong monogamy is how we have to do things?

This book is by no means an attempt to map every single relationship lifestyle. At times it seems like I've taken a reductive approach in grouping relationship types into chapters. Many relationship models overlap and of course each is unique. My investigations merely give a reflection of how we are reshaping our ideals on love and family to reflect a more autonomous and geographically mobile society. Please also note that while gay relationships are relevant to the landscape of modern relationships, I have not dedicated a chapter to them. I've certainly included gay couples in my interviews because they fall into other categories, though. It's my feeling that same-sex unions have been accepted in mainstream society for at least two decades, and this book is concerned with newer, revolutionary ways in which we are conducting relationships.

CHAPTER 1

The Single Gene

When I tell people that I'm in no rush to find a husband, they often reply with some reference to me growing old alone. Usually it's the old lady and cats prosaism. If the alternative to married life was to live in a tank with piranhas I could understand the concern but the cats I've come across have been perfectly harmless, quite friendly in fact. Some people get concerned that I might be lonely when I'm 70. Now I don't wish to sound myopic, but I'm 36! If I were to find a relationship now to ward off some hypothetical state of loneliness when I reach 70, that's actually no less shrewd than buying life insurance.

Anyway, what if the partner whom I take on for my 35-year policy dies before I mature? (Very likely, given that the average life expectancy for women is four years longer than men in the UK[1].) Or he could develop some serious

---

[1] Office for National Statistics

illness and I could end up caring for him. There would be no wild Bingo expeditions and coach trips for me in my retirement years then! Besides, why the pessimism about ageing? I can't imagine octogenarians get lonely these days. They're probably on Facebook organising sherry tastings, or at least they *will* be when I reach 85! Generation Y are children of the social media revolution. Whatever wizened state I'll be in by 2063 (that's when I'll be 85), I have no doubt that there will be a whole sea of never-marrieds, no-longer-marrieds and open-marrieds all flirting shamelessly on the latest inter-care-home dating apps.

I'll tell you another story: the drama of dating doesn't decline with age. One 70+ widower family friend is always telling me about his dilemmas. The last time we spoke there were two women in his life, both in their 60s. There's Lynne, whom he describes as 'wouldn't say boo to a goose' and 'very sweet'. The problem is that he doesn't feel much for her but she 'lets me have sex with her', so he still entertains her. Then there's Kristina, whom he's been taking on holiday and cruises for the last two years and by the sounds of it is totally besotted with. The problem is that she's made it clear that they're never going to get down to any jiggy, insisting on separate beds wherever they go (all at his expense). 'She drives me mad,' he sighed. 'She does yoga and reflexology and all these neurotic things but she is great company, great fun. She has these amazing high cheekbones and is vibrant and full of life. I think I'm in love with her. No, I am – I definitely am. But she's told me she's not into sex anymore. I kept trying at first but I've accepted it now. I still love being with her but as soon as I even go to hold her hand or put an arm anywhere near her, she pulls away because she thinks I'm still going to try to seduce her. But I'm not! The problem is, I can tell Kristina about Lynne because she doesn't mind if I'm having sex with someone else but I can't tell Lynne about Kristina because if she knows I'm going on holiday with a female friend but tell her we sleep in separate beds, she won't believe me.'

You see, all this is to come!

* * *

In the 1950s married couples represented 85 per cent of all households in the UK. In 2012, this figure was 67 per cent according to the latest government figures. A recent trends report by the Office for National Statistics observed that in the 1970s getting married was the most defining part of adult life but today, having children is considered the most significant. How do they know that? Well, in 1971, three-quarters of women were married by the age of 25 and half had given birth. In 2008 only 24 per cent had married by age 25 and less than a third had given birth by age 30. This, the report concluded, indicates that having children has become the biggest milestone of adult life, ahead of marriage.

Fewer people are choosing marriage now than ever before. The official rate is calculated by the annual number of single, divorced or widowed people marrying. Records began in 1862 and up until around 20 years ago the figure for marrying women had remained at around 40–50 per thousand except for the 1940s when it peaked at 63.4 per thousand. But in 2010 there were just 19.8 women marrying per thousand.

To present some figures from another angle, more than 90 per cent of men born in 1930 had married by the age of 40 and 94 per cent of women had married by age 50. Of those born in 1970, only 63 per cent of men and 71 per cent of women had married by those ages. By 2031 the number of 'married' and 'never married' women is predicted to be equal.

Even those who do choose marriage are doing it later than previous generations. The Pew Research Centre reports that the worldwide average age to marry has risen by five years in the last 50 years and is now at its highest ever. In 1960 one in 10 British women aged 25 to 29 was single. Nearly 40 per cent of women in that age group were single by 1998. However, while it may look as if modern youngsters are delaying marriage, the figures are only relative to the last two centuries, when the male-breadwinning ideal has prevailed. In some eras, particularly the Middle Ages, marrying late was common and the average age was mid- to late-twenties.

In her memoir *Committed*, Elizabeth Gilbert visits a tribe in the town of Luang Prabang in Laos, where she finds the elders worrying about an unprecedented problem: the women are delaying marriage. Since tourists started visiting the village, they have been able to make their own money by selling their textiles. Some of them are making use of their new livelihoods and paying to go to college, putting off marriage.

Sociologists and commentators often talk about men and women delaying marriage in a negative light. Even the word 'delay' implies that marriage is still an expectation at some point. But as these examples show, it is inevitable that marriage falls out of favour when a society is afforded greater autonomy.

The renowned Stanford sociologist Michael Rosenfeld identifies a new stage of young adult life that previous generations never experienced. He calls it the 'Age of Independence'. Since the 1960s, middle-class men and women in their 20s and 30s have had the opportunity to live what he calls a 'second adolescence': they leave home and go to college or travel before settling down. He says that this phase of life, which their parents never experienced, is at the root of many social changes. For instance, it means parents no longer have control or approval over who or how their teenage children date. This has spurred a sharp rise in interracial and same-sex unions. According to Rosenfeld, the more a person's relationship deviates from conventional morality, the more likely he/she is to live away from their family. Since we are increasingly geographically mobile, relationships will only deviate more and more from the conventional mould.

The very scholar who established the discipline of sociology, Emile Durkheim was extremely interested in how society was slowly growing to be more independent. In the late nineteenth century he coined the phrase 'The Cult of the Individual' referring to a newfound obsession with one's own life. Gradually, said Durkheim, the individual has become 'the object of a sort of religion, more sacred than the group.' He put this change down to four things: the rising status of women (better education, control over their bodies through the contraceptive pill and more authority in household matters); the communications revolution (the home phone, TV, computers and then mobiles); mass urbanisation (this has created subcultures of single people); and lastly, longer life spans (it's more common for one spouse to outlive the other and then form a new singular life). These four things, he theorised, had created conditions in which the individual could flourish.

So we should not be outraged that full-time coupling is no longer everyone's priority. One thing is for sure, out of the increasing numbers of singletons, there are plenty who are not gazing longingly at their coupled-up peers.

Jake is a 47-year-old single photographer who lives on his own in west London. His last serious relationship ended when he was 34 and for 13 years he has chosen to remain single but enjoys dating. He's funny, good-looking, fit and looks much younger than his years. When I met him he was wearing sunglasses, jeans and a trendy sweater. He was svelte and charming. I imagine he would have no trouble finding a permanent partner, if he wanted one.

'I've not always led a bachelor life,' Jake began confidently when we sat down to talk. 'I was your classic serial monogamist. I came from a middle-class background. Everyone in my wider family had traditional marriages and my school friends have traditional relationships. I followed suit and from 17 to 34, I always had a girlfriend, one after the other. To me single was an interval phase before you met someone else.

'I'd always lived with girlfriends. Not because it was some great romantic gesture but because it made sense economically to rent together. When my last relationship ended, aged 34, it was the first time in my life I could afford to live on my own. I'd never really thought about whether I wanted a relationship until then.

'I felt like I had a blank canvas suddenly and I quite liked the idea of it. I said to myself, I'll stay single for a year, which seemed like a bold challenge. Looking back, I was broadly happy with life when I was living with girlfriends but it felt somehow low-ambition. Like that was the only show in town. Living on my own I had to take responsibility for myself how I spent my time. I started to see how I had blamed my partners for things I couldn't do – in a low-level way. For example, I might say to myself: "Oh, I can't go for that promotion because it would mean moving and I have a partner so I can't". But on my own I couldn't make excuses or moan if things weren't going the way I wanted.'

That was 13 years ago and Jake found he liked his freedom so much that he didn't want to change it – 'I realised single was sustainable. It didn't feel like a temporary state that needed to be fixed.' He continued: 'Now I can't imagine being any other way. If there is something on – an exhibition or an event, I just go. I don't have to wait to see what someone else is doing. I have nothing against people pairing up, it's just that I've realised I don't need that. I'm much happier not trying to fit myself into a template.

'I'd be happy to stay single for the rest of my life but I can't say I won't change and want different things in the future. I can only say what I feel now. I've never felt happier and the casual relationships I do have, have never been healthier. Who knows, I may fall insanely in love with someone and want to be with them every day! It's possible but I can't see it. If someone said, "You can make a deal with the Devil: your life could stay exactly the same. It won't get better but it won't get worse", I'd take it.'

'What are the biggest things in your life that have changed through you being single?' I asked.

'The huge potential for honesty,' he replied without blinking. 'In my previous relationships there were lots of white lies – not dishonesty exactly – but small tactical fibs. For instance I would never say, "God, a hot new girl started at work today". I found myself not saying things for fear that they'd be taken the wrong way. Now I have no secrets with anyone. Likewise, I don't feel anxiety that anyone is lying to me even if it is with good intentions.

'I don't like the dynamic with monogamous relationships that you have to lie to keep things perfect. But I also know that it makes sense to do so. For instance I used to talk to some of my friends about niggles in my relationship that I didn't talk to her about. So there's this person in your life that you're supposed to share everything with but they are relatively clueless about how you feel. That always seemed shitty to me.

'Then there's the fact that I never do anything I don't want to do and I only see people if I really want to. A relationship gobbles up your "grey time". You might say to your partner, "I'm doing this on Monday and that on Tuesday, then Wednesday, no plans". Then someone asks you to go for a drink on Wednesday and your girlfriend is all disappointed and says, "I thought you were free on Wednesday." In a relationship there's a default for your free time and often you end up doing nothing, just being together. And of course the other thing is that I have a varied and interesting sex life – I doubt I'd have that in a permanent relationship.'

'What about children?' I asked. After all, that is the one thing that drives many of us to find a mate.

'I like children but having my own has never appealed. When people see that you're good with kids, they immediately say you should have them. The last person that said that is a horse lover and goes riding often. So I said: "You should get a horse." She said: "I can't get a horse, I'd have to move and I couldn't afford it." Well, children are the same thing! Just because you like them doesn't mean you're willing to change your life and have one.

'Undoubtedly, if I was looking for a woman who could be

the mother of my children I'd be a lot more diligent with whom I dated and find people who only ticked certain boxes. But now I have different people who tick different boxes and I haven't had any problems with that.'

When I tried to track down committed singletons for this book I found very few people identified with this label. After I reframed my search for long-term singletons who aren't bothered either way if they find a relationship, I got far more responses. Rarely does someone rule out love and relationships forever more. It is more fitting to say an increasing number of singletons don't need a relationship enough to compromise with a mediocre one.

Youthful 51-year-old single mum Gemma, for example, wouldn't describe herself as deliberately single, but she's certainly content with her status.

'I'm not single for want of trying,' she told me when we met over a long lunch – Gemma's favourite way to spend an afternoon. 'I've had lots of short relationships but I've always thought there was something better. I got married at 27 and left after 15 months: it felt wrong, I didn't want his children. I thought there was something better out there and I wasn't prepared to settle. I have left lots of people like that, and often in a cold way. I've never dwelled over whether I should leave. There's never been any of that negotiation – I'll change this if you change that. I was always sure of my decisions and I never went back.

'People say relationships need work but I've never been in one that I've wanted enough to want to work at it! Is that right? I don't know. Maybe I expect too much? But I'm happy, there isn't a man distracting me. Whenever I'm asked to do something I never have to take anyone else into consideration. I would find it very hard now to do that. When people say you're too fussy, I think that's not relevant!'

Gemma had her daughter when she was 36. She had been in an 18-month relationship with the father but they split up before their baby was a year old – 'It was a very fateful thing that I became pregnant because if it hadn't happened by accident then I don't think it ever would. I never felt settled enough with anyone to have a child by choice.' Gemma spoke with lots of energy and humour; she was very easy to listen to.

'I left him for the same reason as always: I assumed there was something better. Things were stressful with a young child. I'd gone back to work, he didn't help enough. He forgot my birthday – things like that. We split up, we sold the house and I have been on my own ever since. I wasn't remotely worried how I'd cope: I was the main earner and when he left, I gained control. I like having control of my finances, of where my daughter is, who she's with, how she's getting home. Being a single mum is hard but it is an easier situation to negotiate than being with someone who may let you down.

'I have always wanted a relationship, though. Ultimately we are animals that need mates. After having my daughter, I was looking for the happy-ever-after more than ever because I wanted more children. But it never happened. I've had offers but I've never been willing to compromise my values or those of my daughter. I'd never just settle for someone. If I thought like that, I'd have a man and three or four children by now.

'I gain other things by not being in a relationship. I have far more developed friendships. One friend, who is in a very happy marriage, has invested a lot of time and love into her husband but she doesn't have anywhere near the quality of friendships I have; their focus is each other and everyone else is second.

'I did meet someone recently but the longer you are on your own, the harder it is to adapt. You develop rituals. I ended up doing what he wanted to do to please him. For example, he goes to bed at 9.30 and gets up at 5.30 for his fitness. That's earlier than my daughter! Of course he was happy to leave me in bed in the morning but he expected me to come to bed with him at night. I thought I can never sustain this level of compromise. I see my friends in long-term relationships and they all compromise, so they must want them to work. That's the bit that interests me because I've never felt that.

'I want a relationship in my head. There's a lot to be said for familiar – there's something very comforting about going home to someone who can read you and who you have history with. It's nice when someone knows what sort of mood you're in, or what you need. But I don't want the turbulence of getting to that stage. My life is on an even keel and I'm in control. In the next few years my daughter sits her GCSEs. If I'm going out on dates and thinking of someone else, it's disruptive for her.

'I have to move on from that dream I had as a girl that I'd grow up, get happily married and have kids because the reality is I am grown up and I didn't do it. What I have is no less valuable. In fact, [it's] probably more interesting and rewarding. I'd hate to be in middle-aged misery – a house in Surrey, a couple of old dogs, the kids all gone away to uni and a husband who was having an affair because he finds his wife boring because she gave up a career to raise a family. I'd hate not to be self sufficient and independent. But dreams stay with us and knowing I never realised [mine], does open up a whole load of emotions sometimes.'

William is an even longer-term happy singleton. At 50 he has never married or been engaged. He has had long-term relationships and lived with girlfriends but only because they moved into each other's places, not because they intentionally 'set up home' as he put it. He runs his own small art dealership and lives alone in a studio flat in south London. It's not that he is against meeting a life partner, it's just that he is wary of the demands of living as a duo.

'If I met someone and I was totally enamoured, I could certainly consider a quiet wedding. I just couldn't do the semi and the manicured lawn, and eight shopping bags and the car breaking down and the kids hanging at the bus stop, and the school parents' evening and all that. Quite what I would want from a relationship or marriage I don't know, but I really can't see myself decorating at weekends, going off to Sainsbury's and village fêtes and trimming the edges of the lawn. That is so not me – I can't pretend it could be.

'I think we'd come to an accommodation – we'd have to live somewhere with enough space. You need at least your own room. Not to shut your partner out, but a space you can create as your own. I certainly would need a room filled with books, fresh air and lots of travelling. It's not like I have grand ambitions to do anything world changing but I know that I don't want to be stuck doing something with a wife just because she wants me to be with her.

'I work in a female dominated environment. I like women, of course. I like going out with women, going to dinner with women, but when you've been nagged all day at work and listened to them talk about petty things, I get to the point where I think, "I couldn't go home to another round of that." I'd rather go for a beer with my mates.

'I always imagined by the time I got to 25 I'd be grown up, I'd have a semi-detached and I'd be married and have children. That was what was expected and there was no reason to challenge it. I had my first serious relationship in my early 20s. She was a ballet dancer. She looked like my ideal woman and I looked like her ideal bloke. I always go for the same type – slim and elegant looking. But it was a tempestuous relationship. There was intense attraction but nothing else. She wasn't what I thought she would be, and I wasn't what she thought I'd be.

'We stumbled along for a few years and when we broke up I thought if marriage is going to be like this, I don't want it. She used to say, "It doesn't matter how much people argue or don't get on, it's about the emotional stability." I knew what she meant. There is something comfortable about going home to someone you know: everything is understood, you don't have to explain yourself all the time as you do if you're dating different people. Even if you don't get on, you know where you are. But I thought, "My parents weren't like that – they got on really well, they were good friends." That's what I would want, but I haven't found it.

'I have lived with lots of girlfriends because I thought I needed to for the sake of the relationship. But I've always been better with my own space – I need somewhere to sit and think without someone looking at me. Girlfriends would often say to me, "What's wrong, you look all serious?" I was always perfectly OK, I just needed somewhere to sit and process my thoughts without someone there.

'Do I relish the idea of spending the rest of my time alone? Actually no. I like the idea of having a soul mate. I like the idea that you don't need anyone else and you don't want to be apart, but that's never been the reality.'

* * *

Some people would find the very things that make Jake, Gemma, William and I thrive terrifying for they are daunted by the idea of being alone. Rather than feeling that their identity is eclipsed by a relationship, they need a relationship to prop them up. This fascinates me. I have a hypothesis that there is such a thing as a single gene – a personality trait dictating how comfortable we are operating as single agents.

For instance, why do some women always shop in pairs, yet I simply have to do such functional tasks alone? In my younger days before I lived alone I had a female flatmate who liked to commute into town to our respective workplaces together. She would wait for me patiently by the front door even though I always made her late, preferring my (usually harassed) company next to her than to walk alone. Whenever I see a couple commuting together, I always think, 'What will she do if she wants to pop into a shoe shop en route?' Have you ever jogged with a significant other? Never again! They even insist on having breather breaks together. I know it works the other way too. I'm acutely aware as to how much I annoy my co-sightseers/shoppers/joggers by the number of times I need to pop into cafés and pubs to use the loo. When it comes to functional tasks, surely it's just better to do them alone?

In the BBC Radio 4 show *Desert Island Discs*, interviewees are always asked how well they would cope alone. Some say fine, others – many high achieving, great minds – admit that they find the idea terrifying.

My theoretical 'single gene' is unlikely to be linked to something as simple as confidence or self-esteem because there are many counter examples. Think of former Prime Minister Margaret Thatcher. She had self-assurance in bucket loads but attributed much of her success to her husband Denis being behind her. Then there's Edward Heath, who required similar strength of character to lead a country but remained single, and happily so.

Former glamour model Katie Price hardly needs coaxing to express her self-confidence but she herself has admitted that she's 'not good single'. Yet the milquetoast Susan Boyle, whose brief spell in the limelight terrified her, has never had a man in her life and claims she's never even been kissed!

Susan B. Anthony, one of the pivotal players in the fight for female voting rights in America, was ferociously single-minded in an era when not marrying was unthinkable: 'I declare to you that woman must not depend upon the protection of man, but must be taught to protect herself.' Coco Chanel hardly had an upbringing that bolstered her for tough single-mindedness either. She was brought up by nuns in an orphanage yet rose to become one of the most influential fashion icons we've ever seen, without ever having a man behind her. She had to fend off many questions as to why she never married. 'I never wanted to weigh more heavily on a man than a bird,' she once said. Yet I know an equally strong-minded household-name television presenter who once told me that when she gets home and turns the key in the lock, if she hears silence she goes back out again, such is her aversion to being alone.

In 2008 Swedish researchers from the Karolinska Institutet weren't so far off discovering something akin to the 'single gene'. They examined the DNA of 552 sets of twins, all of whom were in a long-term relationship and had children. They were asked a series of questions about their relationship and their answers compared to their genetic make up. Men with something called 'a 334 version of the AVPR1A gene' rated the strength of their relationship bond lower; they were also less likely to be married. If they were married, they were more likely to have experienced marital difficulties. What's more, when men had two copies of this 334-version gene, it doubled the chances that they would have had a marital crisis in the past year. The scientists concluded this gene could dictate men's willingness to commit.

Professor Cary Cooper is an organisational psychologist and a prolific writer of books on human behaviour and personality typing. I asked him if there are any known factors that make the Coco Chanels, Edward Heaths, Susan Boyles and the Gemmas, Williams and Johns of this world happy with being alone while others are terrified by it.

Roughly speaking, Cooper says, how much we enjoy human contact is down to our personality predispositions of introversion or extroversion. But it's not quite that simple. He describes a concept that he calls 'People Pollution', which can dictate how much we crave time alone. Too much people pollution can drive even the most extrovert socialite to spending time alone. Whether we know it or not, we all have a threshold for how much contact we can tolerate. 'If you go over your threshold you may feel you need time by yourself to reset,' he explains. 'If you get people polluted, you are so overloaded with company, can't cope with any more and need to be alone.

'Today there is more "people pollution" than ever. Not only are our cities becoming denser and more populated, but people's presence invades our consciousness even when they aren't there. We have texts, emails, voicemails, Skype, Twitter, Facebook – we can't get away.'

Professor Cooper didn't even mention LinkedIn, WhatsApp, Bebo and the hundreds of random networking requests I receive. Just this week the little red notification icon on Facebook told me that I was invited to join 'SuperWoman Babe Club', 'Ginger Up Yoga' and 'Performance Platform networking'. I don't even know what these things mean! People continually demand our attention and response. Every time my phone rings, it's another immediate demand. The last thing I'd want is a boyfriend ringing it again, asking for possible dates, five months in advance, for when we can go and stay with some people that I don't even know. After I met the 'proper boyfriend', I noticed how when he received a social invite – Christmas party, summer party, some dull work function, whatever, he'd immediately forward it to me. Can I go too? I had to say yes to at least some of them.

If there is such a thing as a single gene, then we should accommodate the lifestyle choices of those predisposed to it. Just as homosexuals sometimes say they once felt pressurised into heterosexual relationships, there are likely to be thousands of people out there who are way out of their comfort zone with the modern demands of marriage.

Many people who've tried marriage and not liked it would agree. Mark is a high-flying business executive from Edinburgh. He divorced three years ago but remains such good friends with his ex-wife that they live in the same street and share the care of their eight-year-old twins: 'If you want to be married, do it properly and stay faithful but if you don't want to be married, get out! I realised I didn't want marriage anymore. Sometimes I think, was it marriage I didn't want or was it her? I think it was the life. I do worry that I may always be alone but then I think it's only other people that think that's bad. If you don't like the pressures of living with someone, it should be fine to admit that.'

As would Ray, a doctor in his 40s: 'When I was young, I didn't really know what I wanted to do. I just knew that some day I would want to get married and have children, and so I went along with it. I'm glad I've done it: I've got the T-shirt, I know what it's about. But when my marriage ended it was like my life started again – I suddenly got a sense of confidence again.'

Forty-seven-year-old Luke, another long-term bachelor whose brain I picked, was on the verge of marrying and only backed out when given social permission to do so: 'I got engaged at 42 because I thought there was no other option. She was awkward and I had lots of doubts. I was programmed to think that I'd have marriage and kids without thinking whether that was what I wanted; I was sleepwalking into it. It was only when my parents said, "You don't have to have kids for us" that I felt this relief. I then started to question if I wanted marriage either. Perhaps 80 per cent of us are suited to marriage but for the ones who aren't, it can fuck your life up. I thought that I had to find the right girl, settle down and join the marriage club. People prefer it if you're part of the club. Single people are dangerous because we may lead married people astray – we have time to exercise and have hobbies. Married people with kids are dumpy and harassed and have no time for the hairdresser's.'

Psychologist Charles A. Waehler made a similar point while interviewing scores of unmarried men for his book *Bachelors: The Psychology of Men Who Haven't Married*. 'I found that some people have a noticeable ambivalence towards marriage,' he told me when I asked him about his research. 'Those people who don't really want it but go along with it end up withdrawing from their partners or never really engaging to begin with. They may have stood in front of an altar and undergone a legal contract but that's only a marriage by paperwork. That isn't a mature, emotional marriage where they have invested in their spouse. If you want to be coupled go ahead and be coupled, but don't do it just because other people tell you to and then do it poorly.

'We are best as a society when we tolerate different approaches to life but the society we live in heavily promotes marriage. People aren't pushed into it, but it is made clear that coupling makes life easier. You get two-for-one deals on things. The cost of a hotel room is always based on two people sharing. Seats on buses and trains and amusement park rides are usually set up for two. Two people driving in a car will not cost twice the amount of money as two people driving alone. In restaurants there aren't many round tables so if there is an odd number someone goes at the end. There is something functional about the idea of two people doing things together.

'I always chuckle at the idea that it was a premium to be single in your 20s but it becomes a liability when you get to your 40s. What happens to people in these intervening years to make them change? In a crowded room people may tease the bachelor for being single. They'll say, "When are you going to settle down and have kids?" Then the men go into the kitchen privately with them and say, "Don't get married, it's the worst thing I ever did!"'

Waehler's research found no evidence that marriage made

people happier. He followed up his interviewees 10 years later, five of whom had got married, concluding: 'The ones who were happy before they married continued to be happy. The ones who were conflicted and dissatisfied with their lives prior to marriage were exactly the same after marriage.'

Media agency Carat invested in large-scale market research into the single demographic. Its study included 12,000 adults – either single, divorced, widowed, separated or otherwise not in a relationship. When asked what one thing would improve their lives, only one in six of the singletons said 'finding a partner', compared to a third who answered 'getting a large sum of money'. In which case, who cares if money can't buy love? According to this particular study, money is preferable to love.

* * *

With evidence of happy singletons everywhere, it's little wonder we get so infuriated when others try forcing the fairytale down our throats. Whenever common wisdom hints that one has to marry and have kids to be happy, floods of contented singletons jump to their feet to disprove it. In America, strangely more than the UK, there has been a surge of networking groups, movements, talks, meetings and books proclaiming the very pro-single attitude that I exhort.

One of the best known is a movement called Quirkyalone, started by American writer Sasha Cagen in 2003. Then in her thirties she wrote an essay describing how she felt 'deeply single'. She was never in a relationship but she was delighted about it. 'In a world where proms and marriage define the social order we are by force of our personalities and inner strengths, rebels,' she wrote. Cagen estimated that 5 per cent of the population probably felt the same. This turned out to be a conservative estimate because she received thousands of messages and emails from people thanking her for expressing exactly how they felt. Before long she had a website, media interest, a book and was hosting events and organised holidays for thousands of other 'quirkyalones'.

A similarly savvy young singleton Kim Calvert saw a gap in an emerging market and launched *Singular*, a magazine aimed specifically at the professional single demographic in LA. It is now published on the website SingularCity.com. Calvert too believes there are millions of people out there who are better off solo. One of the most popular topics among her readers and her own editorials is the fight to stop single people being seen as incomplete. Another online magazine, Singleedition.com, was started by prolific singleton Sherri Langburt (who is now married). Langburt was inspired to launch the site during her two decades of being single after being riled by a 'join with your spouse and save' promotion for a gym. In an interview with another likeminded blogger of Singletude.com Langburt said: 'I believe that people are just beginning to embrace their independence – it's akin to the start of a liberating new movement. People are more comfortable dining out alone and are excited about solo travel, which was hardly the case during my single years.'

But better than these ideas, a Swedish designer has come up with... wait for it... the *singelringen*. It's a ring to symbolise loyalty to your singledom. Johan Wahlback has apparently sold 200,000 of them to proud singletons in 20 different countries.

I suppose contented singletons like Calvert, Cagen,

Wahlback and I feel we must champion our alternative happily-ever-after moulds because there can never be a benchmark for ultimate happy singledom. No one will ever make nuptial vows to oneself (you can wear the *singelringen* but you can take it off without taking yourself to court). As Gemma, William and Jake illustrate, even the most comfortable singletons are never going to declare that they will stay single forever. This would bind them to exactly the same sort of eternal betrothal that they have so far opted to avoid. A married person can get divorced, so someone who has heralded the benefits of long-term singledom can also get hitched. Romantic statuses are probably best seen as fluid, rather than a pledge we must stick to.

Yet another long-term bachelor I had the pleasure to quiz came up with an interesting alternative to lifelong commitment. Philip envisaged a cultural climate where marriage was not expected to last forever. He had two children from a previous relationship, whom he accommodated at weekends. 'Clearly life-long commitment isn't working for a lot of people,' he said. 'I could never get my head around the notion of forever – it doesn't serve any purpose to lock yourself down. What I propose is a short-term marriage that we can renew at intervals. When I say this to people, they say, "Doesn't that defeat the point?" But I think no, being happy is the point. Maybe if we knew that our marriages were up for renewal every seven years, we might make more effort with them. They say that we change every seven years. My last relationship lasted seven years and I was a very different person at the end of it than the beginning.'

Philip's theory may sound outlandish but not if you consider that seven years is the figure that some anthropologists and evolutionists put on the lifespan of romantic love (more about this later). The fairytale narrative that love should survive the toughest of challenges is so endemic in our beliefs that it seems callous to suggest otherwise. We feel guilty if we fall out of love; like we have no substance if we walk away from a relationship. After several decades, we don't dare admit to our friends that we are no longer sexually attracted to our partners. But imagine if Philip's seven-year proposal was the normal lifespan, if that was incorporated into the fabric of our relationship values. At the end of seven years it would not seem bad or selfish or unusual or shameful to want to move on. In fact the idea that a couple would commit forever would sound radical. It would still be very sad, of course, and some serious consideration would need to be given to sharing childcare, but it might solve the ennui and dishonesty of many marriages.

A seven-year marriage contract seems even less radical when you consider that a third of babies born today are expected to live past 100[2] (that's why I'm buying shares in dating apps for the silver surfers). For a woman born in 1850 the average marriage lasted 29 years. By 1950, it lasted 45 years. Now couples can expect to live an additional 30 years after the kids leave home – an inordinate sentence if you've gone off each other.

One divorcee I interviewed demonstrated exactly how unfavourable this would be. Before her divorce she and her husband had looked into relationship counselling to save their marriage: 'I called up the counsellor first to ask exactly what would be involved and to see if it sounded a realistic

---

2 According to an Office of National Statistics report released in March 2012 called 'What are the Chances of Surviving to Age 100?'

solution. She said, "I can make any two people get on – there is some common ground with everyone." That did it for me. I said thank you very much and hung up. If the reconciliation process was just going to be one big compromise, then what was the point?'

Let's not forget that the choice for us even to assess whether we might have the notional 'single gene' is a modern luxury. Modern life, with all its conveniences, easy networking and high levels of disposable income, leaves little incentive to bed down with a mate for good. Up until the Industrial Revolution, no one could possibly live alone. Few things could be bought ready for use: meat needed to be skinned, fabrics had to be sewn, bread made from scratch and the flour needed grinding and sieving to remove bugs. Put the chores aside, and an extra body was needed simply for the task of grocery shopping. A nifty wife who was good at bagging a bargain could save the family more than she could earn in wages. There was so little disposable income in those days that a day spent scouring different grocery stores for just a penny's difference in the price of individual products might be the difference between three meals a day or two. It just made economic sense to pair up.[3]

As a woman, it has been even more difficult to remain sans husband. For example, when the earliest form of social insurance came into effect in the UK in 1925, it was granted to widowed mothers, not divorced or unmarried ones. Up until the 1950s if a woman fell pregnant outside of marriage, she'd be ushered off to a mother and baby home or in some cases, an asylum. Once she'd given birth her child would be

---

[3] *Marriage, a History: How Love Conquered Marriage*, Stephanie Coontz. Penguin USA, 2006

whisked away and put up for adoption. In *Sinners? Scroungers? Saints? Unmarried Motherhood in Twentieth Century England*, historians Patricia Thane and Tanya Evans cite cases of women discovered in mental asylums in the 1970s, having been incarcerated there for decades and branded 'insane' following pregnancy out of wedlock.

Perhaps it is residual attitudes from the past causing us to continue to favour the couple over the singleton. David Cameron's coalition government has been big on promoting the nuclear family over the single-parent family, introducing tax breaks to married couples but not unmarried ones.

Thankfully, twentieth-century advances in women's rights, contraception and labour-saving technology mean women now have choice. They can marry someone of the same or different sex at whatever age they choose, or not at all; they can have children outside of marriage, in their third marriage or be artificially inseminated by a stranger. All these things can be done without the economic and social disaster that this would have caused a century ago.

Today the strongest factor promoting coupledom is not socioeconomic need as it has been for thousands of years but social pressure.

CHAPTER 2

Everyday Singlism

We single people are like community projects. The most unlikely have-a-go-heroes rise to the challenge to fix us. Willy-nilly, they set us up to any remote connection to other singletons: neighbour, colleague or their cousin's dog walker. Of course if they succeed then it's two singletons cured with one act. Game on!

When I tell friends about a date, they immediately ask if I'm going to see him again before asking whether I liked him. When I answer that I'm not going to see him again, naturally they ask why. I'll say something like 'He was OK but there was no spark' or 'He wears a red anorak and goes trainspotting on weekends'. And they'll say, 'You're too fussy'.

Now this has always puzzled me. 'Fussy' seems to be oddly incriminating to describe the involuntary act of not liking someone. It implies that getting oneself into a relationship is so imperative that the selection process becomes a mere frivolity. It is perfectly OK, of course, to dither over the choice of a pair of jeans, or salad dressing, or the colour of your upholstery. It's fine to be particular about the way you take your tea. It's OK to be fussy about other grave decisions in life – the house you buy, who you elect as leader of the country or who you employ even down to our choice of friends. But when it comes to choosing the person with whom we may end up spending 80 per cent of our valuable free time and disposable income on, who may pass their genes onto our children and whose pheromones will seep into the crevices of our home, we should just be grateful for finding someone. We wouldn't merge two businesses if they weren't right for each other, so why people?

Then my friends will say, 'You just need to give him a chance' or 'Maybe you can get to like him.' As if he's a new job, which I'm stuck with until I find a better way to pay the mortgage. Few can accept that singledom has any sort of durability. To most people it is purgatory and it's assumed that singletons must spend all of their free time doing things that will make them become *not* single.

When I say that I can't envisage having a boyfriend in my life that I have to see every other day, people respond with: 'You just haven't met the right person' or even 'You must want to *eventually*, though'. Or, one of my particular favourites: 'What about when none of your friends are single anymore?' In fact, I fear the opposite. What if my friends *become* single and start organising fantastic holidays to Ibiza and I can't go because I'm on boyfriend-duty. How envious would I be?

Oh, and the most prophetic of all: 'You won't stay young forever'. Because we all know that only the youthful can start relationships. At 50, what are my chances of meeting any of the other 600,000 single men over the age of 50 in the UK, especially with the Internet to help me? I've been reading about a 'new' breed of women called 'swofties' – an acronym for Single Women Over Fifty. The *Daily Mail* has featured several headline-grabbing interviews with swofties declaring what fabulously full lives they lead, 'despite being single'. It's simply radical.

And anyway, it would be a deliberate misrepresentation to marry someone when you know you're on the precipice of decrepitude. It would be like saying to one of my friends, 'That new Mercedes you bought, it won't keep its value for long. Between you and me, it looks like the back tyre may develop a slow puncture and in a few years you can bet the exhaust will come loose when you're right out of masking tape so you better sell it to some unsuspecting buyer now, while you still can!'

There's a disappointing lack of ability to view someone else's framework for contentment with different criteria from one's own. Contentment is seen according to social norms. When a female celebrity says she is enjoying being single the press think it's simply revolutionary. Miley Cyrus, Jessica Simpson, Courteney Cox, Katy Perry and several others have all made headlines merely for saying, 'I'm not looking for a man'.

When my first book *Sugar Daddy Diaries* was published, revealing a passing phase of my life using so-called sugar daddy dating websites, a common question from readers and interviewers was: 'Did you meet someone in the end?' 'Was there a happy ending – did you fall in love?' People are obsessed with the fairytale narrative. There is no satisfactory conclusion to the story until I've left behind my unfulfilling phase of singledom, seen the light and found a man.

Condoleezza Rice gets asked about her love life, when clearly she has far greater things to talk about. Being single hasn't done her any harm: she's become the first African-

American female Secretary of State and later a professor at the Stanford Graduate School of Business. Yet people hone in on her minority relationship status. Chat show host Piers Morgan once pressured her about why she never married on live television. She gracefully swept the topic aside: 'I think I'm well beyond the fairytale marriage stage.'

Cultural references constantly reinforce the idea of marriage as a marker of success. We squeal and say congratulations and we send cards. If someone changes their status to 'engaged' on Facebook, the likes and comments simply go crazy. If you're not hitched by a certain age, you're 'left on the shelf'. Women who don't marry are 'old maids' or 'spinsters'. Actually, if you must know, the meaning of the word spinster only took on a negative slant when the ideal of the love-marriage came along. Originally a spinster was an honourable term reserved for a woman who spun yarn. Later, it took on the meaning of a woman who wasn't married, but it still wasn't derogatory. It was only in the 1700s when we began to aspire to fairytale love matches that it became a bad thing.

Don't get me wrong: I love a good tear-jerking, girl-meets-boy happy ending to a story but a fulfilling relationship should be the cherry on our cakes. It shouldn't be our *sine qua non*.

* * *

In his book *Single: Arguments for the Uncoupled*, English professor Michael Cobb notes 'the contemporary individual is not lonely, just single'. He argues that prevailing novels, movies, TV shows and pop songs depict singledom as miserable and coupledom as euphoric. 'Happy singles are everywhere yet they are marginalised in books and movies,' he writes. 'You can be lonely in a relationship but all those bad feelings about coupledom get projected onto the single person.'

He even goes as far as to say that single people have become 'a hated sexual minority'. Often they take second place for promotions and have no chance of being accepted into high political office. He warns that negative attitudes don't only affect single people but also damage all relationships: 'It is the anxious over-importance of the couple that actually makes couples fail because you can't by definition make a whole world out of one other person. If you try, you're shrinking your world and your existence.'

Harvard sociologist and writer Bella DePaulo first used the word 'singlism' in her book *Singled Out* to refer to the stigmas faced by single people. In America she is the most vociferous force in trying to stamp out prejudices towards those who have opted out of full-time cohabiting relationships.

Cobb and DePaulo are long-term contented singletons themselves and no doubt speak from experience. When I asked my own single friends whether they had encountered single stigma, there was no shortage of responses. I dubbed their snippets 'everyday singlism' because they reminded me of the online project everydaysexism.com, which publishes anonymous tales of women's everyday encounters with chauvinism and sexism.

One friend told how she had recently moved to a new rental property with her two flatmates. She took the day off work and a colleague, fully intending to be sympathetic, said, 'That must be really hard for you – you're in your 30s, still renting and you're not married. It must feel insecure.' 'I thought, "What? I love where I am in life right now." Sometimes I think I should get my own place and a boyfriend, but then I think I only feel like that because society makes me feel like that.'

Another male bachelor friend, who has a teenage daughter he cares for on weekends, said, 'Family and friends always start conversations with, "Have you met anyone yet?" as if that's the most important thing. They don't ask about my daughter, or my work, or my holiday. I can only think they presume that I must be actively looking.'

Stephanie, 41, 6-foot tall with striking looks, is a documentary maker whose work takes her to hostile environments around the world. When I met her through a mutual friend, she had just returned from filming two adventurers trying to set the land record for crossing Antarctica. It was a gruelling trip that required weeks of training. She goes on similarly high-risk shoots every month. Her job has taken her to Afghanistan, Iran, the Niger and uninhabitable jungles. Stephanie has been single 'for as long as I can remember – it just works for me'. But even out in Antarctica she had to put up with everyday singlism. 'The cameraman is married with kids. I was talking to him about how lucky we are that we have the job we have. I've seen some places of the world that no one else will see. I didn't know this guy before the trip and he said, "But Stephanie, you better be careful living a busy single life now because one day you will look back at what you've got and wonder how you missed out." It was outrageous! He totally dismissed my life as less important than someone who is a wife or a mother.'

When I asked Jake, the contented singleton we met in Chapter One, if there was anything he missed about being in a relationship, he replied, 'I miss approval. I miss fitting in.

I miss being respectable. I'm seen as a positively malign force in the world. People think single is a temporary thing or somewhat dysfunctional. It's disordered to not want to find your one true soul mate. There is a narrative that we naturally pair and not pairing is not natural.

'Because I dress normally and I have a good job they are surprised when they learn I haven't had a relationship for 13 years and don't intend on having one. They think I must have been hurt in some way. Weddings are unbearable because people always ask your relationship status. I get the same questions over and over.

'When I have a conversation with someone from an older generation, I always wish I could say I was in a relationship because it somehow implies I'm doing things properly. Single is unserious and not grown-up. Choosing not to share your life is seen as selfish. But then I hear people complaining about their partner, they never take time for themselves and their sex life has died. They complain their life is routine and I think why are you accusing me of being selfish if this is the alternative?

'Some people resent me for having an interesting sex life. You're not supposed to have that beyond 40, you should be concerned with an allotment or something! But then I suppose, if you do something that appears to challenge other people's choices, they can take it personally. It's like saying you don't like a movie that someone likes.'

* * *

If single women are old maids, spinsters, left on the shelf or, to recap author Tracy McMillan, 'selfish, sluts, crazy, liars, bitches, shallow or a mess', this implies that women are the ones desperate for a relationship. If they don't find one, they are tainted in some way. For men, however, the charge is that they must be exploiting women for sex. The most common singlism label for a man is that of the commitment-phobe.

Whenever a high-profile man breaks up with someone who they weren't married to, it's because they are a 'commitment-phobe'. When Hugh Grant didn't stay with the mother of his child, the Chinese actress Tinglan Hong, it was because he was 'still' a commitment-phobe. It was nothing to do with the fact that she was 19 years his junior, from a different culture and the pregnancy was unplanned. When the actor Ryan Reynolds split with actress Charlize Theron after just two months, guess what it was? Reynolds had commitment phobia. (Clearly he didn't because he went on to marry actress Blake Lively.) When HRH Prince Harry turned down a romantic holiday with the beautiful lingerie model Florence Brudenell-Bruce it was naturally because he suffered a 'bout of commitment phobia' according to various press reports.

Celebrity gossip magazines even make top-ten lists of commitment-phobic offenders. George Clooney usually gets number one spot, but Tommy Lee, Jamie Foxx and John Mayer have also been regularly named and shamed. But don't worry, we can banish this dangerous and antisocial condition from the human psyche if we follow a variety of ten steps. Google 'commitment phobia' and you'll get something like 1.5 million results. Scroll through the pages and you'll spot a tireless theme: ten signs to spot it, twenty steps to cure your partner of it, twenty entries of what not to say to someone with it, five possible causes, three women's triumphant tales of how they won the affections of former sufferers, accompanied by happy, smiling photographs of a wedding in the rain.

You can download quizzes to see if you too may be a commitment-phobe. Should you test positive, there are 'homework sheets' for you to complete. You can read a library of self-help e-books, listen to YouTube interviews with psychologists and even book hypnotherapy sessions with commitment-phobia specialists. Quite frankly, this is all nonsense. Commitment phobia is not actually a phobia, not in the clinical sense of the word, which is characterised by an immediate anxiety-fuelled response. If there were such a thing as a clinical commitment-phobe, your date would turn green, get a dry-mouth, hot flushes, vertigo and tremble at the dinner table if you suggested a second date.

Commitment phobia is no more than a convenient label to slap on anyone who isn't in a relationship for any salient reason. The linguistic association with a clinical anxiety disorder shows just how negatively we like to cast those who rebel against the conventional family mould. The phrase was coined in 1987 by the hit self-help book *Men Who Can't Love: How to Recognize a Commitment-phobic Man before He Breaks Your Heart* by Julia Sokol and Steven Carter. The authors 'discovered' the condition, they claim, after interviewing hundreds of men and women on their relationship patterns. 'Our original title for the book was *The Houdini Concept* because it was going to be based on the stories from women of men who act all strong like gangbusters and then back off for no reason. But when we began to interview men about why they act like this, we found that they were describing physical responses – palpitations, states of panic, stomach aches and a sense of doom. One likened the feeling to being trapped in an elevator. That's when we said, "This is a phobia!"' said Sokol.

The authors weren't trying to stamp out this debilitating

condition but merely warn women how to recognise one. They identified two types: the 'nobody is good enough' and the 'claustrophobic' commitment-phobe. The former find fault with everyone so they have an excuse not to commit. 'We interviewed one man from New York who said the reason he had never settled was because he couldn't meet a Jewish woman. New York! It's full of Jewish people, for God's sake!' Sokol illuminated.

Meanwhile the claustrophobics worry about everything that goes with partnering up – 'They are scared of losing their sense of individuality, scared of giving up control, scared of giving up the dream that they will meet their Prince or Princess. For others it is fear of adulthood, fear of dependency, fear of making another mistake, fear of the financial implications.'

But that doesn't sound like a phobia to me. It sounds like the sort of niggles that can be expected from any rational human being when faced with a decision to uproot their life and rearrange it around someone else. Need they have scaremongered men into thinking they could be mentally unstable simply for thinking twice about spending a month's salary on a ring, which has a one-in-three chance of ending up off-set against alimony payments ten years later?

Think about it. Commitment is a pretty overwhelming concept. Here I am, at 36 years of age, having gone through life largely as a singular being. Over the last three and a half decades I have had to somehow muddle my way through learning to walk, my first day of school, picking my first friends, choosing my GCSE options, learning hobbies, my first round-the-world gap trip, university and eventually the bigger choices like a career (I actually had three attempts, starting as an extremely bad accountant).

My whole life it's been me with whom I travelled, me with whom I studied, me with whom I took my first drugs, me with whom I lay in bed while the effects wore off, me with whom I ran up debts and then figured a way to pay them off. Now suddenly, at roughly the midway point, I'm supposed to overhaul all this and accommodate someone else. Suddenly I am to become *à deux*. I will have to think for two, cook for two, book plane tickets for two (and have a big argument about whether we get the early morning flight or the afternoon one so that I can get to the gym). I just can't see it, I can't comprehend it: I don't want it.

Sokol and Carter's so-called 'commitment phobia' may have caught on with the media, hungry for a broad-brush term to explain the demise of every celebrity tryst in *Hello!* magazine but it never caught on in the psychiatric profession. Doctor Lucy Atcheson, psychologist and author of *Anxiety Attacks: Conquering Your Insecurities*, certainly doesn't buy it, 'I don't think commitment-phobia exists solely in the context of a relationship,' she says. 'It's better to call it "fear of commitment" and consider it as reaching beyond relationships. It could have as much to do with commitment to decisions, a career, a mortgage.'

But (and this is the bit I like) fear of commitment is not a bad thing. In fact society needs a few people to have a natural aversion to being tied down because this facilitates cultural change. In the 1940s the existential psychologist and social theorist Erich Fromm developed the idea in his book, *The Fear of Freedom*. He looked at the historical and cultural reasons why most of us find it easier to comply with authority and cultural norms than to think for ourselves. Fromm suggests that we are all born with existential 'givens' – circumstances or traits that we cannot control. Fear of freedom is one of these givens. Fromm observed that many of us go through life subconsciously protecting ourselves from too much freedom because it can be so overwhelming. That's why totalitarian and fascism have been able to thrive in some eras. It's down to those who aren't as scared of freedom to challenge things.

Dr Atcheson applies Fromm's theory to explain why some people are more inclined to commit than others. 'You only need to look at the way we have structured society with laws, mortgages, contracts, jobs and work rotas to see how we manage our fear of freedom,' she says. 'We take away choices from ourselves all the time because as a species we are afraid of too much choice. However, people with fear of commitment have a less heightened fear of freedom. It can actually be a gift because it can open up possibilities that you would otherwise be too scared to pursue. People who take a leap of faith with a move or a dramatic change often have a less heightened fear of freedom.'

That's more like it: a gift. We contented singletons are not selfish, cowardly, broken, desperate or unloved because we'd rather spend our time pursuing interests, careers, friends and shorter romances rather than building a home and a joint life with a partner. We are fearless pioneers, we are revolutionaries, we are love rebels!

* * *

Despite commitment-phobes being stereotypically male, I actually find that it's men who have the biggest issue with those of us declaring peace with singledom. I have a sneaky feeling that men have the greatest interest in preserving the omnipresence of monogamous, long-term relationships. The evolutionist David M. Buss offers an explanation for this in his book *The Evolution of Desire: Strategies of Human Mating*. He suggests that if a man secures one partner, it's his most effective way to guarantee regular sexual access to a female. If he chances it to casual sex, it's a competitive market out there. Women are less willing to play in this arena than in a committed relationship.

Sociologist Eric O. Klinenberg, who interviewed hundreds of single people and people who live alone, for his book *Going Solo: The Extraordinary Rise and Surprising Appeal of Living Alone*, noted nearly all women reported pressure to find a partner and have children. They complained that 'friends and acquaintances constantly drew attention to this area of their life'. The sociologist and stigma expert Erving Goffman once noted that a single woman is not seen for all her individual complexities and achievements but reduced to simply 'the single woman'.

One of the most outrageous examples of singlism I ever encountered came from a man. It was at a friend's 40th birthday. I was sipping champagne, dotting between groups, making new friends and generally having a good time. May I add that I've always found a party easier to circuit alone or with a friend than a date, lover or significant other. Not only are you free to leave early or to stay late as you wish, but a lone ranger seems somehow more entitled to walk blindly into a group of strangers, float in a social sea of new personalities and become scooped into the lottery of random conversa-tions. Going with a boyfriend somehow feels more restricted. There is a behavioural code to follow: you must act as one, include the other, make it known that you are the property of the other. Sometimes, of course, it's nice to have a familiar face to return to when you've had enough of small talk with strangers. But my overall verdict from experience is that there are more advantages going to a social function alone than with a significant other.

Anyway, one such conversation I got scooped into was with Martin, an average-looking single man of 38, with his own shipping business. He had a shaven head and looked fit and well groomed. When it transpired that we were both single he asked which Internet dating sites I'd used. Not whether I was on a dating site, but which ones. At that point in my life I couldn't think of anything worse, which may sound strange for someone who wrote a memoir of a four-year Internet-dating binge. But the thing is, to me there are two reasons why people go looking for dates. They are looking for a stable, committed relationship – someone serious to build and share a life with, in which case the date is a vehicle to get there. Or, they go dating for fun, sexual adventure and to remind themselves how to pull after years of ticking along with someone else. That was me, five years ago. I went online through pure novelty and jejunity, and loved every minute of it. I date hopped between men as I would skip through songs on a CD. I had a dating column called 'Diary of a Commitment-Phobe', in which I sang the praises of my chaotic and highly sexed love life. Friends were in stitches. I collected lovers like dresses. Each was unique and I cherished him in his own individual way, but every so often I'd have a clear out and fancy something new.

Now, I was seeking neither of the above: not a Mr Right nor the exhilaration of a tête-à-tête over a Martini. That's why an Internet dating site would have no appeal whatsoever. If I were to be swayed into a date it would be because I'd stumbled across someone in real life who inspired me.

Trying to manufacture some sort of attraction online would be a bit like eating the bread sticks at a restaurant. Why bother unless you were ravenous?

Between sips of champagne, I tried to tell Martin all this but he was incredulous. He spent the next twenty minutes trying to convince me how important and useful it was to utilise the Internet to meet a partner. The conversation went something like this:

'Why wouldn't you just try it to see if there's someone you like?'

'But I'm not really looking to meet anyone.'

[In a sarcastic tone]: 'Are you one of those career women too busy for a relationship?'

'Doubt it, you're speaking to someone who doesn't start work until noon.'

'But you could be missing out on the person who makes your dreams come true.'

'I might be open to a relationship if I met someone who captivated me but why go shopping when there's nothing you need?'

[In an extra-double sarcastic tone and gesticulating with inverted commas]: 'Captivate you?' *[gives an eye roll]*. 'What if you just got on?'

'I have lots of occasional lovers that I "just get on" with.'

'*Lovers?* What about when you get old and your lovers lose interest and you'll be all alone?'

And so on.

I once went out with a man who tried to convince me that I needed to find a husband when we fizzled out! I should mention that this man, Jason, was one of my so-called 'sugar daddies' in my said former life. He was a travelling American businessman and so I only saw him four times a year while on assignments to Europe. It was a convenient set-up: I would travel in style and be put up in fabulous hotels and, because he could afford it, he would take me on extravagant shopping sprees. We were never going to be anything more than travelling lovers. He was 20 years my senior and although I'm reluctant to admit it, he was married but his overseas girlfriends were an open secret.

While Jason may have enjoyed his temporary inamorata, he made it very clear that at some point I should forfeit our temporary relationship and seek a permanent partner for myself. I think he considered this to be honourable, selfless advice but it was downright irritating.

'You really need to find a rich husband,' he would say.

'What on earth would I want one of those for?' I'd laugh. But he found my frivolity insincere: 'What is your alternative, if you never get a boyfriend? You'll be an old lady with no one to care for you.'

I'd give him the usual response: how I liked being single, how I thrived on independence, how women now earn their own money and how my busy nature is not the type to ever fall short of fulfilling things to do.

'Everyone needs a life partner!' he would exclaim with urgency.

'Why?'

'Because we lack the inner strength to get through life on our own.'

'But what about someone who is independent and doesn't feel they need to lean on anyone?'

'Not possible!' he cried. 'A woman needs a man to get

through life, and a man needs a woman. Tomorrow you will have an epiphany and you will thank me. Show me one person at 60 who is alone and happy. You need to open yourself up to meeting someone. Life is about the long haul and you have to think about the future. At 40, you won't be so beautiful and then what will you do?'

He even said twice that if his eldest son wasn't already married he would try to match-make us. Imagine! Also, he couldn't understand me not wanting children. When I said I found them boring, he would dismiss me as 'not understanding the joy!' 'Boring is good if you want to create a stable life. You'll see,' he insisted. I found it so infuriatingly patronising.

Perhaps I should not have been so surprised. After all this was a man who took no shame in admitting that he married his wife for money, was encouraging his daughter to marry a man for money and was in the process of persuading his second son not to marry a girl who had no money. Despite this admission, he reminded me repeatedly how much he loved his wife. He talked of her fondly but also complained constantly about irritating she was, how she nagged and how they had stopped having sex years ago.

I once asked him why he loved her. His response confirmed my theory that we often manufacture our own feelings because it suits our needs. 'Because she's the most efficient person in the world,' he replied.

'Is it her or the relationship that you love?'

'OK, you got me!' he threw his hands up. 'It is the relationship, I admit that but I do love her. She keeps me in check and she makes my life easier.'

I didn't disbelieve that he genuinely loved his wife but he did so because of how she facilitated his life, not because he loved the essence of her. That was why he was having an affair. He claimed to love me too but that was also because I fulfilled a role: I was his mistress abroad.

Being a recovering alcoholic, back home in the States his family and friends prevented him from drinking. In a secret compromise deal he struck with himself, he allowed himself the luxury of drinking only when travelling. 'It makes abstinence a more realistic prospect,' he told me. And drink he did! He took in vodka martinis virtually intravenously. We hardly ever had sex. Well, we tried a few times but he always drank too much. He wanted me not for a sexual encounter but as his drinking buddy in feminine form – a sympathetic, soft, sensuous figure to accompany him in his guilty vice. 'I just love the company of a woman,' he once told me when I asked why he had always sought affairs even though he adored his wife.

As an object of desire, I was planets away from his stable wifely figure back on the West Coast. Like many men across many cultures throughout history, he distinguished between the two roles. He exercised his drive for romantic love with his lustrous mistress and his drive for deep feelings of attachment with his caring wife.

If you think about it, most people have a self-serving reason for sticking with a relationship, whether or not they admit it. Perhaps they want children so they speed up their search. Maybe they don't want to work and they meet someone perfectly tolerable but not electrifying, who can support them. Or they just want to fit in with the lifestyles of their peers. When I asked a selection of people what it was about a permanent relationship that was so appealing, one woman said, 'the dream of a country cottage with children in dresses and a rose garden.' Another man told me, 'I like the idea of having a base. There is a security in that. Knowing where you are, knowing that someone understands what's going on in your life and you have someone to run things by. It makes me feel like I belong somewhere, like I have roots. I feel more secure about everything in a relationship – my decisions. I like to know that I have someone behind me.'

Another man, a widower, who had just got together with a new partner, said that the thing he appreciated most was that 'she found things for him' when he constantly lost them – 'She's just brilliant. She looks after me.' The same man reflected with brutal honesty that he had never really loved his wife. Their wedding, at 18 years old, had been encouraged by their parents and was 'the right thing to do in those days'. Yet even though he didn't love her, he said he 'missed her terribly – we were a team. We shared the house, the children, the dogs… Being a couple is just neater. When we travelled somewhere we had the surname and a joint bank account. We booked rooms for two, seats for two, dinner for two. I resent her going because I've got everything to sort out on my own.'

Our self-motivated reason to find a relationship is often so subliminal that we don't even notice it. Every long-term committed relationship I've had, I can trace back to an event or time when I had a need for someone in my life. I met one boyfriend 10 years ago, following the death of my father. Before him, I had just moved to London: new city, no friends. Previously, it was my final year at university and I couldn't stand the mouse-infested, damp and musty house I lived in or my insomniac party housemates. I wanted to be out of there as much as I possibly could, and guess what? I happened to find a man with his own mini-flat in his med school quarters.

Of course I felt genuinely in love with these boyfriends at the time but that does not discount the fact that I, like everyone else, made an unconscious calculation of the benefits and losses in pursuing a relationship. For those who enjoy constant companionship, there are lots of ticks for being in a relationship. But for those with the metaphorical single gene, the benefits are scant.

In her book *The Best Kept Secret: Men and Women's Stories of Lasting Love,* Professor Janet Reibstein made the same point. She interviewed hundreds of couples to try and uncover the so-called 'secret' of lasting love. And what did she find? Not selfless love, but hard-headed utilitarianism. 'Almost every relationship, consciously or not, is based partly or wholly on parameters such as domestic practicality, financial security and parenting duties,' she told me. 'People who romanticise their lives more might not notice the pragmatics of what draws them to their partner but it becomes more conscious over time as their lives become more intertwined. Once you start to share your decisions on holidays, how much you spend, where to live and then managing children, you start to realise the compromise you've made. If you're the one getting the rough end of the deal, you start to recognise it more prominently as a trade-off and can feel resentful.'

All this suggests that long-term singletons like me – the so-called 'commitment-phobes' – are more romantic than those who constantly chase love. It actually makes serial monogamists seem disingenuous. Contented singletons stumble into love because they find it, rather than hunting it down because they can't live without it.

If ever I have that epiphany as premonished by Jason, or I 'meet the right person', like my friends foretell, then I'll definitely go for a self-sufficient commitment-phobe. With a steady serial monogamist, I'd always suspect it was the company he was after, and not me!

CHAPTER 3

Man Not Included

On my run to the gym every morning I pass a small bandstand in a park. Often there is a group of about twenty women with puffed cheeks pushing prams in a funny trot in circles, round and round the bandstand. Always one or two are under the gazebo in the middle, tending to a soiled baby on his back screaming so loud it sounds like a band's in action. This is the local Buggyfit class. Every time I jog past I think, 'Please God, don't ever let me be one of them!'

Hold on, before you start drafting that hate mail! I have nothing against Buggyfit mothers or their Fit Momma sisters, I just wouldn't want to be speed-walking with a pram myself. The reason why I suddenly take to praying that I may not become one of them is because there's still a part of me that thinks child bearing is beyond my control; it is something that I will one day have to woman up to and do.

Like many women, I've gone through my whole life thinking having children was something that would happen in the future – after marriage maybe or when I'd got my career to a satisfactory level. Perhaps when I'd got London out of my system and moved to the country. I thought the moment would arrive when it would feel right to have them. That moment was always in the distant future. As I got older I realised that I had put that moment in the distant future because I didn't want it ever to arrive. It had never occurred to me that I might be able to choose not to have children and it was only when I took a close look at this elusive 'moment in the distant future' that I thought, actually I'm happy sticking with the moment that I have, thank you very much.

I now know with 99.99 per cent certainty that I do not want children. It's quite a simple neural process which tells me what I like and what I don't like. The same, I imagine, that lets me know that I prefer Italian to Chinese, that I don't like Marmite and that I secretly enjoy the soundtrack to *Dirty Dancing*. But it's amazing how many people think that they know better than me about what I like. I must want children *really*, I just don't know it yet. Of course I'll want them 'one day'. Or perhaps I just 'haven't met the right person yet'. (This right person, by the way, has a lot to live up to – I've heard so much about him!)

I am a woman, I must want children; I should be a natural at raising my voice three octaves and speaking that way for four years and making aeroplane shapes with plastic spoons of liquefied carrots.

Some people find a woman who says she doesn't want children disturbing. I once went on a date with a (divorced) man who said that a woman who doesn't want children is not a real woman. I swear it's true. He hadn't seen the irony that his own marriage had ended because he grew tired of his wife after she gave up her entire career to look after his children and their beautiful five-bedroom home with five acres and as such, only ever talked about the latest release of Monkey Music and what flavour cupcakes she ate while waiting for baby yoga to begin. He had an affair with a more exciting, independent, freethinking, childfree, younger woman, got caught, and she kicked him out and kept the family house.

I know many single men who say that they would not start a relationship with a woman who doesn't want children. That's a good thing! Men need to take an active interest in whether they want a family, rather than rely on their girlfriend's 'natural instinct' to kick in. I know one man who dismissed his girlfriend when she said she didn't want children – he presumed she would one day change her mind. When she didn't, he started to gently pressure her. Five years later, still no mind-change from his girlfriend and so eventually they broke up and he found someone who did want children. I'm sure the severity of the broken hearts on both sides might have been reduced had he taken note of his broodiness earlier.

Female public figures that haven't had children are often vilified. Australian former Prime Minister Julia Gillard was once described as 'deliberately barren'. Dame Helen Mirren has told of how she has repeatedly had to explain why she chose not to become a mother. In an interview with *Vogue* magazine in 2013 she said the pressure wasn't from women: 'It was only boring old men. And whenever they went "What? No children? Well, you'd better get on with it, old girl", I'd say, "No! F—- off!"'

Some people even get angry with women who express their wish to remain childfree. I received abusive emails on an Internet dating site from two men because I'd ticked the 'I don't want children' check box. I 'shouldn't be looking for a relationship' if I wasn't interested in bearing a man's child, apparently! Oh, and I'm 'selfish'.

Selfish? Why, because my genes are so superior that by not breeding I'll deprive the world of the person who's going to solve world peace, come up with the next generation of penicillin, devise a replacement for oil or stop the jet stream ruining our lovely British summers? Sorry, I'm just going to leave it to one of the other 700,000 babies born each year on our sinking, overpopulated island to sort out. I'm *so* selfish!

Oh, and the other one I've had is: 'It's a crime if you don't have children'. Naturally I'm flattered – but a *crime*? Who's the victim? Some unborn soul stuck in purgatory in need of an infant human body to anthropomorphise into?

In her memoir *Turned On,* Lucy Dent, who wrote under a pseudonym, described how she visited an online mother's forum and typed in: 'I don't want children, is there something wrong with me?' She was met by a stream of outraged responses from angry women calling her a disgrace to her gender and accusing her of taking her womb for granted, and other insults.

If a woman doesn't sacrifice her life in some way to someone else, to mother, to smother her love over her children or her man, she is unwomanly. Cold. Non-maternal. Non-nurturing. Yet if a man decides not to have children, he's just 'independent' or 'too focused on his career' or he 'didn't meet the right person'.

I get the odd passive-aggressive comment – 'Having children is the most rewarding thing you can ever do' – but most people simply allay my fears with an attempt at empathy. Their responses usually start with, 'How old are you?' And then they give a knowing nod because at my tick-tocking age of 36, there's still a slither of a chance that I just haven't discovered my maternal side yet. Then they say, 'I didn't want them either but I fell in love/I hit 38/my hormones kicked in/once they're born, you won't feel like that'.

They say all these things with an 'I-know-better-than-you' expression on their haggard, sleep-deprived faces, which isn't the best advert for their cause. I'd rather collate my own evidence to make my decision on whether I want children or not. One only has to look around. Restaurants at weekends, car parks at national parks, the seats at the front of economy class of any flight, a few clicks on Mumsnet ... All these are incredibly effective modes of contraception.

People tell me that 'the love you feel is so overwhelming, it's all worth it' but I've also heard as many women say, 'If I'd known what I know now, I may not have had them'. One man (another date, I'm afraid – it's a great life-shaping hobby) made this point beautifully: 'The love you have for your children is so powerful. If you could bottle it, it would be like concentrated euphoria. But it wouldn't be something you could use in large doses. It would be like perfume, you'd just take a dab of it. On a day-to-day basis, they're a pain in the arse!'

One other protest against popular wisdom I would like to air is the assumption that broodiness kicks in when the urge to get drunk and dance on tables until 3 a.m. fades. I can attest – I've had more than generous lashings of unruly behaviour in my time but these days I'm more likely to be listening to *Book at Bedtime* on Radio 4 with a herbal tea than doing any of that. But in no way has my new interest in my health and sanity ever translated as being ready for a baby.

In *The Whole Woman*, Germaine Greer writes: 'To become a mother without wanting it is to live like a slave, or a domestic animal'. If I ever got struck by lightening and woke up maternal, I would either watch an episode of *Bedtime Live* or take a short trip to the countryside to stay with my sister, brother-in-law and my lively nephew and niece, now aged five and three, to instil some sense back into myself.

One particularly traumatic visit stands out. It was a cold summer – the type where everyone insists on eating outside even though it's drizzling and there are 30 mph winds – because it's *summer.* The youngest, then one, had just learned to walk; the eldest, then three, had just learned the negotiating power of tantrums. The family house was being renovated and so they were temporarily living in a cottage at the end of the garden, which meant I had to shack up with the three-year-old at night. He chattered in his sleep all night – total gobbledygook with his eyes shut. Admittedly it was very endearing...

...for the first two hours.

Then it started to feel as if I was hooked up to a Linguaphone tape of an Inuit dialect. He woke up a few times horrified at this blonde thing in his room that looked a bit like Mummy but wasn't his real mummy and burst into tears.

The second night I slept on the sofa.

I love them very, very much but oh, the chaos! Breakfast was out of the question. There were toys to fetch, juice demands to deliver, toast pelting to manage, potty training bloopers to see to and rescue missions to extract something from the one-year-old, who kept finding new and dangerous objects to put in her mouth. Reading a newspaper seemed like a luxury experience for the elite.

When I tried to wash up, my niece cried. I picked her up,

her bib drenched in a mix of snot, baby milk, purified carrots and dried sick. Then I walked around, mumbling some nonsense in what I hoped was my three-octaves-higher comforting baby voice until she calmed down. Just as she started to smile at Aunty Helen, my sister appeared from her shower, spotted the plastic bowl carnage at the sink and said, 'Helen, haven't you washed up?'

Then the eldest one, sensing that the adults had diverted their attention away from the train tracks he was building onto each other again started to tug on Mummy's dress. Mummy picked him up and told him that Auntie Helen would play with him. Meanwhile Aunty Helen's porridge was still in the microwave.

Another time, when the youngest one was very tiny there was one day when the poor little thing had a tummy bug. She kept being sick… again and again. We were out in the garden and there was regurgitated milk over everything. Just as I thought she could be sick no more, I picked her up and she was sick again. All this milky pink fluid started to trickle down my *décolletage*. I asked (well, maybe I *shrieked*) for my sister to hold her so that I could go and wash it off. She looked at me as if I was more neurotic than Howard Hughes and said, 'It's only *baby* sick. Rub it in!'

Rub it in!

This is a common theme. Mums simply dab wee, sick, poo, snot and grubby fingers and say 'never mind'. It's as if the body fluids of babies are made of spring water. I constantly see mothers sniffing their babies' bums to see if they need changing. It's completely gross but because it's a baby bottom it doesn't count.

Even the dads are affected. I once watched in horror as my brother-in-law calmly walked over to my niece and wiped her runny nose with his fingers and then, while he was there, he picked out a limey green gooey bogey from her nose and casually rubbed his fingers together once completed. I let out something that sounded like 'irrrrrr!' To which he looked at me in a oh-you're-such-a-clueless-city-girl kind of way and said, 'It's only a *baby* bogey!'

Another childfree friend (this is the last anecdote, I promise, and it's a good one) relayed her own horror story at witnessing her sister place her mouth round her 18-month-old son's blocked nose to suck out the snot. She then spat it into a tissue and said cheerfully, 'There, that's better. He can breathe again now. Poor little thing!'

That's love! We will see in Chapter Five just how obsessive romantic love is. But if romantic love makes us go nutty, maternal love is positively psychotic! I'm surprised it hasn't been classified yet. '*Mother-psychosis*: [**muh***th*-er-sahy-koh-sis]: Characterised by delusional beliefs that one's offspring are cleverer/better looking and more advanced than anyone else's; Uncontrollable desires to update Facebook with daily photos of one's offspring; Has compulsions to talk obsessively about offspring, often failing to recognise facial disinterest in one's speaking companions'.

By not wanting to embrace maternal love, I am far from deviant. In Britain today one in five women over 45 is childless. That's not so different to the 1920s when 23 per cent of women remained childless. For the latter it wasn't because they wanted to lead hip, globe-trotting, childfree lifestyles, it was more likely due to extreme poverty, poor nutrition and low marriage rates because of war. Today it's the wealthy who are more likely to be childfree. Across Europe the figure for childlessness remains at around 20 per cent but rises to 50 per cent among females in senior levels of professional or managerial jobs. In Sweden, where there is lots of access to childcare, it is 12 per cent.[4]

In her research for her memoir *Committed*, Elizabeth Gilbert concluded that in every human population the world over, the number of childless women has always been at least 10 per cent. Many times and places it has been much higher but, she claims, never lower.

Gilbert suggests that this constant 10 per cent-or-more figure is evidence that Nature intentionally retains a supply of childfree women. The world needs them, she argues, as spare child carers for when it all gets too much for frazzled mums. Or for when war or famine strikes and some of the mothers are wiped out. Gilbert calls childfree women the 'Aunty Brigade' because of the care and attention they are able to give other people's children. She presents them as unsung heroines. Florence Nightingale, for instance, was able to put her unused nurturing capacity to good use in hospitals. Others like her have been able to run schools and orphanages. The Aunty Brigade often steps in with financial help for nieces and nephews when their parents' purse strings are overstretched.

It may not sound like it, but I love being an aunty. I may not be good at sick trickling down my *décolletage* but I do look forward to offering them my love and support throughout their whole lives. And I can't wait to earn my stripes as the cool aunty who gives sage advice. I love following the development of my friends' children – I find it fascinating when I see a friend's characteristics personified in mini form. Parenthood is a significant part of adult life so it

4 'Childlessness in Europe' (Report for the Economic and Social Research Council), 2005 Catherine Hakim

would be antisocial and unsustainable for the childfree to ignore it. Me, I'm still perfectly willing to take part in the Easter egg hunts and games of rounders in the park; I just don't want a family of my own.

Children are hilarious and offer a window into the raw human condition. They're affectionate and, when they're not covered in snot, I've been known to find one or two of them cute. But boy are they boring! And between you and me, I've always found the smell of babies makes me feel a bit sick.

If I were a man, I think I'd quite like to have children. Despite the glory given to the modern hands-on dad, men still bear nowhere near the same burden as women. Dads are the advisors, the entertainers and the fun ones. A father's role is more satisfying and less stifling than a mother's. It's not just the obvious physical burdens of pregnancy and labour: a woman is predisposed to feeling a far stronger sense of maternal responsibility. If a man walks out on his family, it's bad. When a woman walks out, it's shocking. Men can claim diminished responsibility.

It doesn't escape me that not wanting children plays a huge part in my attitude towards relationships. If I did want to raise a family, it's certainly easier to do so with a man who's pledged his life to me and is willing to share his income.

So what happens when women become mothers without a man? Does the urge to find a permanent partner simply go away because it's mission accomplished already? From meeting many of them, I would say that it does.

* * *

In a large Mexican restaurant in Chelsea in west London one hot Sunday in August, a group of around thirty women, mostly in the early- to mid-40s, gathered for lunch for their annual summer social. The prams and pushchairs and bobbing female heads made them easy to spot when I arrived.

I introduced myself and squeezed into a seat in the middle of the long oblong table packed between two unsmiling women. It looked as if most of those around the table were already well acquainted.

'What's your name on the site?' demanded one auburn-haired, slightly overweight woman in her late 30s.

There was an awkward moment as I replied that I wasn't 'that active on the site' and I was there to find out more. As I spoke I could almost see a barrier rise between us. I was an outsider. If I wasn't active on the site, how could I possibly contribute today? How could I have any idea of what the women here were going through?

The site she was referring to, which linked all the women at today's lunch, was fertilityfriends.co.uk, a forum for single women looking to have children through sperm donors.

Like Gemma, who we met in Chapter One, these women had put to bed any fairytale aspirations to meet a perfect partner and create a family but had instead set about carving their own family set-ups, something incomprehensible just 50 years ago. The woman's defensive reception gave me a jolt of realisation at just what an emotional ordeal it must be to make this decision.

It was hardly surprising that someone turning up out of mere curiosity would be greeted coolly. Unlike me, the women around this table longed for a child. They had probably watched on painfully for years as friends and colleagues got hitched and became pregnant. Almost certainly, they were startlingly aware of their ticking biological clocks, feeling an extra pang of urgency with every monthly cycle that passed. They may have grimaced at the costs and physical discomfort of their fertility treatment and had to overcome fears of facing pregnancy and child rearing alone.

On the discussion threads of fertilityfriends.co.uk the most common topics are how women coped with the difficult decision to go it alone, the challenges of single parenthood, the costs and successes of different insemination techniques, concerns about explaining to their future children how they were created and the sadness that none of their friends could ever understand what they are going through.

I sat down and tried to absorb as many of their stories as I could. Around half of the women had already had sperm donor children and were keen to offer support and advice to those following in their footsteps.

I had first contacted the organisers and asked if I could attend the gathering as a researcher. My request was ignored so I joined the website forum and went as a paying member. However, once there I felt awkward infiltrating such a deeply personal soul-sharing session and using it for my own research – like a medical student rummaging around a corpse. So I came clean and told them that I was writing about sperm donor mothers and would they mind if I listened in and absorbed. Thankfully they were delighted.

'I'm happy to get the message out there that we will be much better mothers than a lot out there who don't even want their kids,' offered Bibi, an attractive Asian woman.

She was 11 weeks pregnant but as she put it, 'not silly enough to uncross my fingers yet.'

'I'm 37 and to be honest, I've been broody since I was 27,' Bibi relayed, and there was a murmur of agreement around our section of the table. 'I was in a relationship but although he said he wanted children, he didn't. I have had other partners since but none of them seemed to match my need for children. I always thought, if I get to 35 and I haven't had a child, I'll have one no matter what my circumstances. When I got to 35, it wasn't like I thought, "Oh shit, I have to do it now!" Instead it was a relief – I didn't have to wait for the man anymore. It took the pressure off.'

'Have you ever thought that the relationships you pursued in the past had more to do with wanting a child than being with them?' I asked, thinking for the third time how glad I was that I had confessed my research role because I would never have been able to ask such a probing question otherwise.

'Totally! Suddenly the rush was off. I used to look at every single guy and think, "Could it be you?" but I'm not even looking at guys anymore.'

'I had a similar thing,' another woman called Penny, 43, added. Like many of the women there she hadn't made much of an effort with her appearance. She had wiry greying hair and no make-up. Not that that has a bearing on her likelihood of becoming a mother, but it perhaps symbolises her apathy for winning the attention of a male now that she has a sperm bank to provide for her. 'When I made the decision to go to a fertility clinic, a relationship stopped mattering. Obviously it would be nice to meet someone, but this [fertility treatment] is my focus now.'

'I don't try to make relationships work like I used to,' said a smiling girl called Rebecca – the most cheerful I met that afternoon. Everyone was incredibly serious. She looked younger than Penny and also appeared to have skipped on grooming. She'd brought along her six-month-old son, Charlie. 'I've got into Internet dating recently but it's just for fun and to be honest, it's great to have sex again!' There were sniggers around the table. 'I don't want a man in my house all the time. It makes me feel good to have a bit of attention but it's not like I'm looking for a father for Charlie and I never let them meet Charlie. When I told my mum what I was doing, she said, "You'll be better off in the long run. You don't have to worry about someone else's dinner or what he wants to do."'

This point obviously roused the group because I could hear the drawing of breath as they queued to add a point. 'I have a friend who recently split up from the father of her child. She says things are much easier. She said he was like having a second child,' said one.

Another added, 'When I was voicing my concerns to my friends about how hard it might be to go it alone, the predominant response was that their husbands don't help anyway. There is a common sentiment, muttered under the breath of women everywhere, that their husband is more of a hindrance than a help.'

'When I read things in women's magazines like "get your partner to rub your feet at night in your final trimester" or "pump some breast milk and get your partner to do one feed in the night", I think, yeah, right! When I ask my married friends if this really happens, they laugh. I've got one friend whose husband slept all the way through his paternity leave.'

Another sperm donor seeker Anna, who I met independently of the networking lunch, articulated this even more strongly. At just 32, she described herself as 'not the type to keep a partner'. According to her she is easily bored and easily irritated and thought it better to go it alone:

'Any relationship in recent years has been in view of having a child. I don't want to waste time with the wrong male when I could be spending time with a baby.

'I got pregnant once with an ex but had a miscarriage. He didn't seem to care about it. That shocked me. It was so huge to me I couldn't comprehend his indifference. I think I pushed him away after that. Then I was in a relationship with a guy who couldn't have children. We tried IVF. It didn't work and we broke up through the stress of it all. That's when I thought: do I want a relationship so desperately?

'You can waste time falling in love. I wasted so much emotional crap on these guys. Years ago I was engaged to a guy who was really awkward – I was give, give, give the whole time. If you have a child, it's give, give, give too, but at least you know what to expect and get something from it. With him I got nothing but grief.

'I'm not looking to date any more – I've done that, been to great places and had lots of fun. I can have that again some day but I can only have a child now. This seems like the most straightforward way of getting to where I want to be.'

If a man were to listen to women like Anna or to read some of the postings on fertilityfriends.co.uk, he might well develop an existential crisis: 'I know a lot of people will say I'm quite young to be going it alone but I don't really want to do this with a boyfriend,' wrote one 24-year-old on the online forum. 'I decided to go it alone when I found myself in a crap relationship. It was great to begin with, we both wanted children, but eventually I realised he was just saying that to keep us together,' said another. 'Ideally I'd rather not do this alone. But if it's a choice of relationship or a baby, the baby wins any day.'

There are several options for an immaculate conception. The cheapest and crudest form of artificial insemination is via a home insemination kit – they can be bought from the Internet for around a fiver. All you have to do then is find a willing sperm donor. That's easy because there are now lots of sperm donation websites to choose from. They work a little bit like a dating site: donors and recipients post a profile, photograph and message each other. When a woman finds a donor she likes, she can either invite him round for coffee and he can masturbate into a pot in her bathroom or he can send it in a custom-made chilled, vacuum-sealed vial by courier right to her front door. For this, the sperm donor asks a measly £50 for his 'expenses'. Which means, in theory, a whole life can be created for £55 – less than a dinner date.

But with this budget option comes risk. Sperm donor websites are unregulated by the HFEA, the watchdog that oversees storage and use of gametes, and so the recipients won't know anything about the quality of the man's sperm or whether he has been screened for hereditary conditions or sexual diseases.

The other way of doing things is to go through a licensed fertility clinic. Obviously it's much safer but eye-wateringly expensive and time consuming. Each cycle of artificial insemination can cost up to £3,000. The most common form of artificial insemination for the clinics route is IUI, which involves a laboratory procedure to find the fast moving sperm and place them in the woman's womb during ovulation. The more expensive and more complex IVF procedure is when eggs are removed from the ovaries and fertilised with sperm in the laboratory.

With donor sperm from a licensed clinic, by law the father has to remain anonymous until any resulting child reaches 18, in which case the child can decide whether he/she wants to learn the identify of his/her father. However, when a woman opts to use 'fresh sperm' from an anonymous donor website, it's up to the individual and her donor to agree whether or not the father stays anonymous, which opens up all sorts of risks.

There is another less talked about method of sperm donation gaining popularity on sperm donor websites. It is euphemistically referred to as 'natural insemination' or NI. Which is – yes, you've guessed it – real sex. Many women advertise for 'natural donors'. Several men will respond and once the woman has found one she likes and trusts, they will arrange to meet while she is ovulating. I once went undercover on a sperm donation website to write about NI for a national newspaper. It was quite clear that most of the men were not offering their services for altruistic reasons. Sadly, most saw it as a fantastic opportunity for one-off unprotected sex, rather than the chance to help women create life, as they claimed.

Saying that, there are many men who also wish to procreate for procreation's sake. Many men on donor web-sites are spurred on by the prospect of posterity, but they want nothing to do with changing nappies or watching nativity plays. I once interviewed a very nice guy called Steven, a 42-year-old divorcee with two biological children who live with him full-time. For the past 11 years Steven has been donating sperm continuously – through sperm banks, online fertility forums, donor introduction agencies and even via his own page on Facebook.

He makes at least two donations per week. Women travel to him from all over the country. Sometimes he has to drop everything and fly abroad at the behest of an ovulating woman. He has 26 sperm donor children that he knows about, but thinks there could be as many as hundreds more because he doesn't stay in touch with most of the women he donates to.

Sometimes the women pick up Steven's sperm specimen from his home. Occasionally he meets them with it in a pot at a service station. Or if his recipients really want to stay anonymous, they send a courier. He was incredibly laid-back about it – almost jovial. He lives a clean life, drinks rarely and works out every day; he doesn't mind whether or not the women want him to have contact with his children. All he asks is that the mothers sign a form to attest that they won't chase him for child maintenance payments. He's happy to visit on birthdays and Christmas if required but equally to disappear if that's what the mother wants. He says he loves the thought of his 'gene pool being out there', spreading and multiplying throughout the population.

I believed him. Since he charged just £50 for his efforts and £20 for each subsequent sperm pot in the same ovulation cycle, he certainly wasn't doing it for the cash. The women do pay his travel, though, and he once visited Brazil so it can't all be bad!

Anyway, rather than saying that men are being made redundant by test tube conceptions, it's more accurate to say that romantic relationships are becoming less relevant in the arena of procreation.

I should make it clear that the women in the Mexican restaurant that Sunday afternoon weren't anti-man. Nearly all of those I spoke to pointed out that starting a family without a loving partner would not be their first choice. The reason they were doing so was exactly the same reason as Gemma (Chapter One): in today's climate there is no need to compromise with a less-than-satisfactory relationship.

'It devastates me that I have to do it this way but I couldn't live with myself if I thought that I hadn't at least tried to conceive,' said a softly spoken, slim woman of around 45. 'There is no one that I can talk to about it. Friends can't begin to understand what I'm going through and it annoys me when they can't see how seriously I take this. I get mood swings with the fertility drugs. My family worry that I won't cope as a single mum and try to discourage me. I can't go out drinking because that disrupts fertility anyway so I just stay at home.

'This is why I don't like the term "single mother by choice". I am not single by choice – I will be a mother by choice, but why would I choose to go on this stressful journey alone with miscarriages, crazy hormones and the expense?"

'I'm happy being called a single mother by choice,' piped up a small, smartly dressed girl with a neat, dark brown bob. 'I'm pretty Zen about opting out of the marriage thing but not about the mum thing: I *have* made a choice.'

Her name was Anne and she was only 30, already a successful family lawyer in Leeds and five months pregnant through IUI. Conservatively dressed, she had not a hair out of place. She spoke slowly and clearly, appearing totally in control.

'In my job I see so many unpleasant disputes over access to children, day in, day out. I see parents arguing over Christmases and birthdays, right down to the last hour of time they can spend with them,' she told me. She had a calm, considered style of speaking.

'I've always longed for children. I was a nursery nurse before studying law – I loved it. It was becoming more and more difficult seeing other people with children because you want what they have so desperately. Eighteen months ago I was diagnosed with ovarian cysts, which had to be surgically removed. My ovaries were saved, thankfully, but I heard that the procedure can affect your fertility so it shocked me into doing something. I visited a clinic and I knew straight away it was for me.

'I started to see that a relationship would have been a means to an end. Any relationship I have had, I've always tried to accelerate things so I could have a baby. It was the same pattern, history kept repeating itself. It wouldn't have been fair for me to stay with any of them. I said to myself, "I don't want a relationship that isn't meaningful just to get a baby from it." So I decided to go ahead on my own.'

At this point our main courses arrived. The most gigantic cheesy enchilada and big fat chips were placed in front of Anne, in stark contrast to her prim turnout and collected poise. 'Eating for two!' she laughed.

Another woman standing over us, winding a tiny baby on her shoulder, asked whether Anne felt just a hint of a craving for a boyfriend now that she was pregnant? 'Didn't you want someone to share the first scan or the first kick with? It's never as interesting to your friends and family as it is to the father. Most of my friends just smiled and went "That's nice!"'

'I do crave love,' resumed Anne, taking all the attention in her stride. 'But I've never met the right person for that. I was conscious that love may not come along until it was too late.'

'From all the divorce cases you've dealt with, do you

think there are any two-parent relationships that can last?'
I asked.

'I do,' she said with her mouth full, but somehow still
perfectly composed. 'But they are not the majority. Children
end up stuck in disputes and they can become badly damaged
by that. Some people think I am selfish but I have seen other
children affected by growing up in a hostile environment. I tell
people that what I am doing is more responsible. I'm in control
of everything my child will see – no one else.

'One friend asked whether I had considered my child if
something happened to me. I was furious. Of course I'd
thought about it! Any mother – in a relationship or not –
lives in permanent fear as to what would happen to her
children if something happened to her. That shouldn't stop
you doing a wonderful thing like giving life.'

This opened a new and equally popular topic – guilt over
the unconventionality forced upon their unborn child. What
questions would their children ask? How will their little
minds process how they came into the world? Why does
Mummy not even know Daddy? Was there never a daddy
who loved them, or even who loved Mummy?

'The thing that gets me is not knowing *anything* about his
father.' This from the woman with the baby on her shoulder,
who was now falling asleep on a muslin. 'How do I explain to
him that I know even less about his father than a one-night-
stand? If I just fell pregnant after a night out, I wouldn't
hesitate in going ahead with the pregnancy. But going through
a donor took up so much thinking time. I worry how he'll cope
with it. I plan to tell him as soon as he's old enough but I know
he'll go straight to school and blurt out to everyone in the
playground that his dad's a sperm donor – I dread to think
what the other kids and mums will make of it.'

Perhaps these reservations and concerns show just how strongly the link between love and procreation has been imprinted on our consciousness. First comes love, then commitment, then a baby from *natural* intercourse. That's what the fairytale marriage narrative teaches us. But for these women, love and commitment hadn't come along at all. A prince was not the lead role in their fairytale. For them the most important plotline in their happy-ever-after was having a child.

* * *

There are currently two million lone parents in the UK, an increase of half a million since 1996 according to the Office for National Statistics. In some parts of the country, such as the urban areas of London, Liverpool, Manchester, Birmingham and Leeds, single parents outnumber couples. Britain has the highest proportion of children brought up in one-parent families of any major European country. Twenty-three per cent of 14-year-olds grow up in single households. The only other country where this is higher is America, where it is 26 per cent.

Unlike sperm donor mothers, most single parents don't set out to be single parents. In fact there are just 800 babies born from donated sperm in the UK each year according to the HFEA, and even then not all mothers of sperm donor babies are single because sperm donation is also popular with infertile or lesbian couples.

Statistics show that around half of single mothers were married when they had children. Only 6.5 per cent of births are registered by one person and another 10 per cent are registered by two parents who live separately; only 8 per cent are single dads.

Over the last 10 years, the numbers of parents bringing up children alone hasn't increased that much, though. ONS figures show the biggest rise was from 1970 (when it was only 8 per cent) to the late 90s when it reached 23 per cent and since then it's only crept up. But like declining marriage figures, there are many who argue that the rise in lone parenthood is a sign of a fragmented society (yes, *that* argument again). Government social policy experts have long proffered that children need input from both parents in order to thrive. The bulk of research does indeed show that youngsters growing up in fatherless homes are less likely to do well at school and more inclined to get into drink, drugs or crime, but just as many studies show that love and attention are more important than whether two parents are present.

Entering parenthood alone isn't ideal. The average cost of raising a child to age 18 is said to be £146,000, according to a report by Child Poverty Action Group. Other commercial studies such as one sponsored by insurance firm LV put the figure even higher, estimating the cost of seeing a child to their 21st birthday at £222,000. Not all lone parents are affluent, emotionally mature professionals like the women at the fertilityfriends.co.uk event, who can afford thousands of pounds for artificial insemination. The less glamorous reality is that 48 per cent of single mothers are unemployed.

Added to that, there's no one to babysit if you want a night off or to allocate the school run to once you're back at work. No second income to fall back on if you're made redundant. But it would be preposterous to argue that having the choice to become a lone parent is a bad thing. Thank goodness having children no longer chains two adults together; that the stigma around lone parents has subsided enough so that men and women don't have to resort to a stilted co-existence with a half-hearted monosyllabic spouse in order to raise a family.

Three decades ago, you wouldn't hear a woman say: 'I realised I was only with him to have a baby and that wasn't fair so I decided to go it alone.' Up until the last few decades, getting married because you were having a baby was the right reason. The shotgun wedding was the best option for any woman who unexpectedly stopped her periods. Whether her inseminator was Mr Right was irrelevant.

Today women consider the challenges of single motherhood and lone pregnancy a much more agreeable compromise than the emotional drain of a disconnected relationship. As the women I spoke to repeatedly paraphrased: 'This wouldn't be how I chose to do it but it's better than an imperfect relationship.' What these pioneer sperm donor mothers demonstrate is that partnership these days is worthwhile only if it promises significant love and true compatibility.

CHAPTER 4

Relationship Revolution

'So me and Sarah have both banned them. They can't go.' My friend Hazel slammed her oven door shut and looked up at me with a triumphant expression.

'Is the stag a close friend of his?' I asked. I was sitting on her worktop, shelling a bottomless basin of organic peas, my shoeless feet dangling on the work units, watching and listening as she simultaneously cooked a casserole, packed a lunchbox, stripped a set of rain-sodden clothes off one of her sons, answered the phone three times and talked to me. Now I watched her throw ingredients into the dish aggressively. She was relaying a... let's say... exchange of opinions between herself and her husband the night before.

'They went to school together,' she replied. 'But he's bad news. Loads of the guys on the trip are single so they'll be a bad influence. It's tough, he's not going!'

I was visiting an old school friend in my hometown that I hadn't seen for perhaps a decade. It was strange to see the girl who was once my clubbing companion standing in a ginormous kitchen, apron on, surrounded by carrot peelings, with the distant sound of children's voices from various ends of the five-bedroom house. Hazel met her husband when she was 18. As I was packing myself off to university, she was planning her wedding, pregnant with her first child. Now that child was preparing university applications and there were two more roaming around the house too.

She had hardly stood still for the two hours I'd been there and every task I'd watched her do seemed to be laced with resentment. Her husband, a steady and loyal local chef, was supposed to be going to a friend's weekend-long stag do in Amsterdam, much to Hazel's protests. When I asked why she said, 'Because he might get off with someone.' 'Getting off' being our northern colloquial slang for snogging a stranger in a bar.

She was no longer a close enough friend for me to comment but what I wanted to say was, it's this sort of deprivation that makes being married feel like a sentence rather than a pleasure. This sort of rule setting will make him want to reassert his individualism in some way elsewhere.

In four years of writing about relationships I come across cases of what I call 'couple control' wherever I go. I see men who have to abide by so many rules and routines to keep the domestic peace that it makes a totalitarian regime look tame in comparison.

Just a few days before shelling peas with Hazel, I was at a journalists' networking event, where I talked to a young freelance writer. She was excited because she had just secured her first full-time magazine job. It started in two months' time, which meant she was about to give herself a long sabbatical.

'I was going to go to India for two months but my

boyfriend wasn't keen on that idea,' she told me. 'He said he'd miss me and he worried I might forget about him, so we compromised and I'm now going for two weeks.'

Now perhaps I've been single for so long that I've forgotten the default obligations felt when you are part of a couple, but I couldn't see any sense in this at all. To me, it seemed a pointless compromise to her sense of self. Unjust even. And for what and why? I remember thinking how horrible it would be to be in a position where a rare opportunity came up to utilise two wonderful months of work-free time, only to have it whipped away because of boyfriend-bureaucracy, to live in the constant presence of potential veto. No matter how much I was in love, I thought, I'm certain that I wouldn't forfeit a once-in-a-lifetime extra-continental travel opportunity unless I was satisfied that it served some logical purpose. Nor would I try to restrict the person I loved.

I often hear people joke about 'getting permission' from their 'other halves' to do things. In my pre-freelance journalism days, when I worked in an office, I would hear colleagues in the pub – male and female – joke about being in trouble if they got home late. They'd plot to 'sneak in a quick one' lest they be reprimanded for getting home too far past bedtime. (Is their partner afraid of the dark?!)

If there were nappy changing duties to attend to fair enough, but I see many perfectly perky twenty-somethings dragging themselves away from a pumping party so they can go home and pretend to enjoy rubbing their partner's feet while watching *Casualty* with a packet of Doritos. I remember a row with an ex once because he'd been away for work for a week and instead of meeting him at the airport for some grand celebratory homecoming as he expected, I went to a university reunion with friends that I hadn't seen for five whole years and probably wouldn't see for another five. This clearly didn't align with his views on how I should have prioritised my time.

Last week, I listened to a young couple on the Tube arguing for about twenty minutes because (I think) he didn't want to go to her friend's party that night. 'What are you going to do instead?' she demanded to know. It was clear that he didn't want to do anything, he just didn't want to go. Why make him? I thought. My mum's friend drags her retired husband around shopping malls every Friday afternoon. He loves walking and the outdoors but she wouldn't be caught dead in a Barbour or a pair of wellies. It's not that she's short of friends to take shopping, it's just that she can't bear to leave him home alone. She says she's worried what he might do. Heaven forbid he might make himself a cheese sandwich and leave crumbs!

While we're on this subject, may I just point out how frustrating it is when women insist on bringing bored-looking boyfriends and husbands to the shops with them. It's not just tedious for the blokes, it ruins the experience for the rest of us. The men follow their girlfriends and partners round like monosyllabic teenagers, sneaking in a text or checking the football scores and blocking up the aisles for the real shoppers!

But I digress. Another overheard conversation in a café recently between two men revealed that they were attempting to co-write a screenplay but one of them was struggling to find a window to do so: 'I try to do an hour every day when I get home. I don't always want to, but I tell myself just an hour,' the first one said.

'I wish I could do that,' replied the second man. 'But my

wife gets annoyed because I don't relax with her. Even on a Saturday morning, I wake up at 7 a.m. but she *makes* me lie there and says we should lie together.'

My sister tells her husband off for finishing the leftovers. He tells her off for having another glass of wine so she pours it while he isn't looking (she's going to kill me for that one). Of course they do it for each other's own good, but they're grown-ups. They censored their own behaviour perfectly well before they met.

Another acquaintance I know is positively resentful of his wife. He calls her 'the witch' in front of his friends, much to their amusement. Also, he makes jokes about the jobs and tasks he's been given and the things he's been 'told off' for. He drinks to oblivion and then stays out for as long as he dares as an act of rebellion. Sometimes, he tells me, he deliberately uses the wrong set of crockery to the one she tells him, 'just to annoy her'. I asked him why he behaves so destructively. 'Because I'm on a leash,' he replied.

So why this stamp of ownership, why this forced duty? I imagine a lot of it, like a boyfriend who insists on picking his girlfriend up after a night out, or the wife who demands her husband comes home by a set time, is down to jealousy and fear that their partner might be unfaithful, but I can't think of anything more likely to drive a person into someone else's bed than control.

In the few long-term relationships I have found myself in, of course I've had episodes of irrational fear that they might be attracted to someone else. Like anyone else, I've lain awake in bed and thought, 'What if he's having a wild blow-out night and he's met some girl? What if he's dancing nose-to-nose with her, right now? What if he's having sex with *three* women right now?' But there is no point in worrying about this. You may be able to suppress someone's actions with curfews and travel bans but you can't suppress their urges. There will always be someone prettier, wittier, younger, more successful, more intelligent and more interesting. All we can do is hope that the partner we love doesn't want to chase, sleep with, love or have threesomes with anyone else because they are totally enamoured with us!

Another undercover journalistic mission of mine was to go on a marital affair website for a newspaper. I posed as a married woman looking for an affair – complete with fake wedding ring and everything. I'll embellish on this mission in a later chapter, but the crux of it is, when I settled into conversation with my dates and asked what had driven them to join a cheating site, every single one said that they still loved their spouse but they had an urge for new, fresh, exciting romance. I loathed their sense of entitlement and their cold, calculating approach in using a website to deliberately manufacture an affair. But I did learn that in their minds what they were doing was nowhere near as malicious as their wives would have considered it to be. To them it was an outlet for their physical and adventurous fantasies and it didn't detract in any way from the deeper love they had for their partners.

It may be hard for most women to comprehend, but if a man happens to have an opportunistic marital blip it's not so emotionally threatening as they may think. A one-off fling isn't a patch on the feelings they have built up for their long-term partner over time. I now think that the male predilection for fresh sexual experiences is so deeply entrenched that it's better to try to understand and accept it than to control it. Tagging is just fidelity under duress. The only thing that makes a man or woman stay faithful to the person they love is their own will.

The well-known celebrity divorce lawyer Vanessa Lloyd Platt has advocated what she calls a 'marriage-lite'. She described it as something which 'should involve respect and companionship but absolutely not taking each other for granted. It shouldn't be about picking up each other's socks.'[5]

I think I could handle a marriage super-skinny extra-lite. Someone to love and to hold tight, though not every single night. If modern relationships did not require such intensity, I might be tempted.

* * *

This whole fairytale aspiration of modern marriage – that our partner should be the fabric of our life and the core of our happiness – didn't originate in the days when we lived in monastic castles and knights rode around on horses anyway. The idea of finding a soul mate and living happily ever after is new – 200 years new, in fact. Comparative to the 10,000 years of civilisation, that's not very long at all.

Up until 200 years ago, marriage was for securing beneficial in-laws, increasing the family labour force, bettering political ties, creating business partnerships, securing trade deals, gender division of labour, furthering social status, acquiring wealth or bettering one's living standards. But it was rarely about love. If the couples involved did happen to be in love, it was incidental.

In a crude attempt to summarise the complex and multi-

---

5 *Dangerous Women: The Guide to Modern Life*, Clare Conville, Liz Hoggard and Sarah-Jane Lovett. Weidenfeld & Nicolson, London, 2011

layered history of marriage in the Western world, I'm going to start by setting the scene 12,000 years ago, at around the start of civilisation in the region of Mesopotamia, along the banks of the Tigris and Euphrates rivers, in what is now Iraq.

My summary here, by the way, relies heavily on the excellent history provided by Stephanie Coontz in her highly readable *Marriage, A History: How Love Conquered Marriage*. Our Stone Age ancestors lived in foraging hunter-gathering societies, sharing all their resources – food, shelter, sexual partners, you name it. They had no privacy, no personal property, no favouritism. Women breastfed each other's babies and everyone relied on each other for protection, companionship and food. Both sexes hunted and gathered. They formed alliances not in cosy twosomes but big clans. The bigger your family, the safer you were because it served as your protection. Although couples formed within these clans, and formed the basis for breeding, most researchers believe couples dissolved and reformed much more easily.

The closest thing they had to a ceremonious marriage was an exchange of men or women between groups because they knew this was genetically advantageous.[6] Some anthropologists cite evidence of group sex, lesbianism and a regular exchange of sexual favours. There was nothing taboo about this – this was communal living after all. Then along came the agricultural revolution, somewhere around 7–10,000 BC. People clocked that dividing land and cultivating crops in groups was far more economical than individuals going out to

---

[6] *Sex at Dawn: The Prehistoric Origins of Modern Sexuality*, Christopher Ryan and Cacilda Jethá. HarperPerennial, London, 2012

forage every day. That, according to the anthropologist Christopher Ryan in *Sex at Dawn,* 'changed *everything.*' Land could now be possessed and passed down to children. Food that was now shared had to be harvested, stored, bought and sold. Fences and irrigation systems needed to be built and armies were needed to defend it all.

Large-scale clan-like communities were no longer practical. People took on individual roles and that meant a more rigid gender division of labour. Previously, men hunted large animals and women foraged or engaged in small-scale hunting, but there was lots of flexibility. Now, women needed men to plough, men needed women to weave blankets, preserve food and to bear children to provide and care for them when they grew too old to work. Some historians go as far as to say that monogamy itself has its routes in the agricultural revolution. The notion of 'owning property' gave men the idea that women too could be owned – one woman for every man.

It isn't clear when or who invented marriage itself – some attribute it to the ancient Romans – but the concept of permanent pair bonding, whether they had a ceremony or not, was cross-cultural after the agricultural revolution. Gradually the agriculturalists started to migrate and expand their communities into towns and villages. They formed villages along the Tigris and Euphrates, claiming more and more land until they formed kingdoms and then dynasties. As civilisation grew more complex, the differentiation of wealth magnified and social hierarchies emerged. And that's when the motive for relationships changed again: marriage became not just an important tool for a livelihood but a weapon to seize power.

Social rank was everything in those early days, so it was

highly beneficial if you could lay claim to noble blood. What better way to do so than to marry into it? Marriage became a highly strategised procedure to further family ties. Families would offer their sons and daughters to wealthy families. If needs be, they'd negotiate further by throwing in a few fields or work animals. Men of lower classes would offer themselves to princesses or daughters of a powerful family, sometimes bringing their own slaves and workers as part of the deal.

Those already high up in the kingdom stakes needed to surround themselves with a trustworthy network as protection. Rulers and noble families used marriage as a means to retain power by choosing spouses whose families offered valuable diplomatic, military and commercial connections. Sometimes there would be a case to marry their children off to an overseas family to secure a base on foreign shores. Stephanie Coontz compares the large families of this era to the powerful corporations of today, and likens marriages to important business mergers. Roman aristocrats she says, would 'divorce and remarry as freely as changing a mobile phone contract'. They simply switched if they found a better deal elsewhere.

So much was at stake through marriage that it became a battleground. In the upper classes it was fraught with brutal rivalry, feuding and betrayal. It wasn't uncommon for a mother to plot the murder of another woman's son if she wanted her own son to have dibs on a particularly eligible young lady. Or for the new husband of a high-ranking widow to try to get rid of the sons she had with her late husband in case they posed a threat to the new family line.

Selecting a partner was so important, so strategic and so

consequential that it was not left to the individuals themselves. Relatives, neighbours, judges, priests and government officials all got involved. Personality profiling was the last thing on anyone's checklist! Some outspoken individuals tried to manipulate their own matches but even then, it wasn't often for love. They had their own ideas on who would bring them the best political or economic gain.

Among the lower classes there may not have been so much power or inheritance at stake but marriage matches were still done to benefit the couple's families. Who you married rested on whether your in-laws would be beneficial connections, their fields were strategically positioned next to yours and what labour skills your spouse could add. As Coontz says, '[Marriage] was too vital an economic and political institution to be entered into solely on the basis of something as irrational as love.'

Of course people still fell in love in those days and many couples were in love when they married but this would have been a bonus rather than a necessity. Some cultures did indeed encourage marital love but I imagine only in the same way as a boss may encourage his team to bond. Moralist commentators of the sixteenth and seventeenth centuries, for instance, reassured apprehensive women heading into marriage that if both sides 'are of good character, love would follow'.

Even when couples were in love, it still wasn't acceptable to place love above more important issues like kinship or business agreements, or feelings for God. Across the world the most significant relationship was considered to be between birth relatives.

In ancient India love before marriage was considered disruptive or antisocial. In China, men who showed interest in their wives were considered weak – grooms could be beaten by their fathers or brothers for siding with their young wives. In ancient Roman culture it was considered disgraceful to kiss one's wife in front of others. Greece too joined this sentiment, referring to the sin of loving one's wife as 'adultery'. Catholic and Protestant theologians referred to spousal love as idolatry – the sin of valuing something more than God. Churchmen scolded wives who used affectionate nicknames for their husbands because it undermined the man's authority. These political motivators for marriage remained the status quo for thousands of years all the way through to the Middle Ages and beyond. And yes, even during the beginning of Christianity.

Most of us think that 'holy matrimony' was a virtue of the early Christians. But no, while the blood-thirsty murders and intrigue of the ancient dynasties may have calmed down, in biblical times people still saw marriage as something which secured business networks and inheritance rights. When Jesus Christ came along with his teachings of Christianity, he told people it was better to remain celibate and organize one's life around the church than to marry. The heart should remain firmly with God, he taught: 'If anyone comes to me and hates not his brother, mother, father, wife and children and his own life, he cannot be my disciple' (Luke:24). It sounds dramatic, but what he meant was that you have to give up an awful lot to be a true believer. So unless you relinquish alliances to family and spouses, your heart will be too divided to be a serious follower.

Marriage wasn't exactly discouraged by Christianity but it was considered a second-best alternative. Saint Paul instructed divorcees and widows to refrain from settling down again. In Corinthians 7:8 he says: "I say to the unmarried and to widows that it is good for them if they remain even as I." Christians, you see, believed that purity of the soul was the ultimate achievement in life and since marriage involves sex and sex is impure, marriage was also considered impure. (But then, if you consider that early Christians continually thought the world was about to end, you can see why family building would be the last thing on their minds.) [7]

Despite these Christian teachings, people still married – they couldn't form important business and family ties unless they did. In fact they took marriage into their own hands, getting hitched whenever and wherever they liked. They didn't need deeds, signatures or witnesses; they got married simply by declaring themselves married. Over time, people adopted a little more formality to wedding ceremonies and started to use witnesses, but not for the sake of romance. It was to avoid arguments over whether the two parties had consented to marriage in the first place, in case they divorced and there were disputes over land and property.

Yes, divorce. Society was far more forgiving of divorce in the centuries prior to the Middle Ages than we are today. But something happened in 1215 to change that, something that made marriage a life sentence mostly to the detriment of women.

Royal courts, noble households and aristocracy were becoming increasingly powerful (mainly due to all their strategic marriages). This concerned the Roman Catholic

[7] *Committed: A Skeptic Makes Peace with Marriage*, Elizabeth Gilbert. Bloomsbury, 2010, UK

Church and so, in 1215, it made a move to control matrimony by outlawing clandestine marriage. Suddenly all marriages had to be under church supervision. Then it banned divorce, except under Church approved annulments, which would be issued when it suited their purpose. This effectively made marriage inescapable – catastrophic for a woman with a bullying or violent husband. It remained the law until 1533, when Henry VIII quite spectacularly reintroduced divorce. He wanted a divorce so that he could marry his lover, Anne Boleyn. Defying the Pope he ordered the Archbishop of Canterbury to grant him one. (Incidentally, this act of love rebellion contributed to England breaking away from the Catholic Church.)

Marriage didn't remain fluid for long, though. In the eighteenth century a popular legal doctrine known as coverture spread through Europe, putting married women in a straitjacket again. Under the laws of coverture a husband and wife were seen as one person. The concept of coverture emerged in the Middle Ages but it wasn't codified into law until the eighteenth century. The wife's legal existence effectively disappeared: she couldn't own property, file lawsuits or execute contracts. If she went into marriage with property her husband could use, sell or dispose of it without her permission. And he couldn't leave any property to her when he died even if it was hers to begin with.

Coverture was arguably one of the biggest blows to women's rights in history. Marriage by definition eradicated all rights, freedoms and personal property of a woman. Residues of its oppressiveness remain in customs and laws today. It was because of coverture, for instance, that women in some states of America could not take out their own loans until 1975. Also, up until 1984 New York State still recognised a marital exemption in its rape laws.[8]

But back to the 1700s. It was shortly after the laws of coverture became ingrained in English common law that young people got it into their heads that they should marry for love. Among those rebels to societal mores was the poet Samuel Pepys when he chose to marry 14-year-old Elisabeth de St Michel.

In the mid-eighteenth century Gretna Green became a refuge for love rebels. The town was just north of the Scottish-English border. A law was passed in 1754 in England stating that anyone under the age of 21 who wished to marry needed parental consent. The Act didn't apply in Scotland so in-love couples sneaked to the border to make their vows.

The idea that one should marry one's sweetheart was a seismic change in the history of marriage. Behind it were two things. First, the Industrial Revolution of the late 1700s introduced waged labour. Servants and manual workers could be paid with cash rather than food and accommodation. This meant young people no longer had to stay with their families and wait to inherit land or a business before marrying. Nor did they have to live with extended families after they married.

Second, this was the period of Enlightenment. People started to believe that human relationships should be organised by rationale and justice, rather than force and birth right. Power struggles ensued. People wanted to choose their leaders, their religion and their profession;

---

8 *Committed: A Skeptic Makes Peace with Marriage*, Elizabeth Gilbert. Bloomsbury, 2010, UK

they started to talk about happiness as if it were a legitimate goal in life and so of course, they began to talk about seeking happiness in marriage and emotional fulfilment from their partners. It may not sound a big thing now but the pursuit of happiness was made a right in the American Declaration of Independence, an über-radical idea at the time.

But everyone was concerned about the idea of a love marriage. If men choose their spouses for love, surely women would demand a say in household decision-making? If relationships were based on mutual affection, why would women submit to domesticity?

Women worried too. Would men still stay with them if they fell out of love? And would they still provide for their wives if they couldn't discipline them? Conservative commentators muttered that this pursuing happiness lark would disrupt moral order. They predicted that it would lead to a rise in divorce and leave a trail of broken homes and a tidal wave of legal disputes over wealth and possessions.

And guess what? They were right! As Elizabeth Gilbert wrote in her own summarised history of marriage, *Committed*: 'Everywhere, in every single society, all across the world, all across time, whenever a conservative culture of arranged marriage is replaced by an expressive culture of people choosing their own partners based on love, divorce rates will start to rocket. You can set your clock to it. It is happening in India right now'.

It was this tsunami of change in attitudes that gave rise to the fairytale marriage. When, in 1850, Queen Victoria walked down the aisle in a flamboyant white wedding gown, accompanied by music, the public was mesmerised.

No one had known such a custom before. Overnight, weddings became ceremonious affairs, decadent celebrations of love.[9]

It was also during this era, marriage historian Stephanie Coontz notes, that people began to embrace the excesses of romantic love that previous generations had warned against. People wrote love letters to those they wished to marry; they talked about being forlorn without their loved ones. Literature embraced flowery love stories.

The fairytale had formed.

* * *

They didn't know it but the Victorians were guinea pigs for a revolutionary new societal trend – they were the first to make married love the centre of their lives. But it wasn't all happy endings. Far-fetched romantic dreams to meet a nearest-and-dearest drove many people not to marry at all because they feared that their high expectations for a soul mate would not be realised. Novelist Catharine Sedgwick was one such romantic spinster. She wrote that she had recurring nightmares about marrying the wrong man and in the end she married no one. Evidence again that those with the 'single gene', the 'self-centered' commitment-phobes, are just too romantic to settle.

As the fairytale ideal of the love-based, happily-ever-after marriage set in, so too did new ideals for femininity. Women in the 1700s were career-orientated but young women of the next century were encouraged to stay at

---

9 *Celebrating the Family: Ethnicity, Consumer Culture, and Family Rituals*, Elizabeth H. Pleck. Harvard University Press, USA, 2000

home, protected and provided for by their loving husbands. Gender stereotyping helped solve some of the problems that the new love-based model of marriage threw up. For instance, confusion about who held authority in egalitarian relationships was solved by the presumption that men and women's roles were so different that they couldn't possibly encroach on each other's territories. Men went to work and got involved in political affairs. Women stayed at home and put their efforts into making themselves and their children as aesthetically and educationally sublime as possible.

By the mid-1800s the recipe for Utopia in the middle and upper classes became the male-breadwinning, love-based marriage. The family became the nucleus of society. Men were praised for putting family duties ahead of business or social arrangements. Wives were cast as fragile and pure, blinkered to any expression of sexuality whatsoever, resulting in the reticent sexual attitude for which the Victorian period is so well known. In reality, it was only the more privileged classes who could afford for the wife to stay at home, practising the piano and pandering to her *toilette*. For most, the Victorian dream was unattainable. Rich families used it as an excuse to berate the lower classes. Any woman who did not stay at home was clearly not dedicated to her family and therefore unrefined. Middle-class women would hide the fact they had to work. Male-breadwinning family status was a marker of class, much like having kids who go to private school or a holiday villa in the Algarve.

But this was not to last. The offspring of demure Victorian mothers had other ideas. Middle-class women were starting to attend high school in growing numbers so their appetite for life stretched beyond the home. As the economy prospered, new roles emerged for secretaries and typists and assistants. Experience-thirsty women snapped them up. Office life meant socialising with men and it wasn't long before the Victorian custom to mix in separate gender circles faded away and a dating landscape allowing natural affections and compatibility emerged.

It was the women of this era who started the Suffrage Movement of the 1890s. This would change gender relations forever. Women who had previously been groomed to be wallflowers embraced the fight for personal expression and political clout. The more aggressive mouthpieces of the movement slandered marriage as a form of oppression. Men were scared. Some alarmed opponents argued that giving women the vote would lead to social revolution, disruption of domestic ties and desecration of marriage.

Meanwhile there were all sorts of new and exciting things available to the adventurous youth – dance halls and cinemas and motorcars – all of which granted them privacy, much to their parents' horror. Alcohol and cocaine were easily attainable – social lubricants which no doubt helped the Roaring Twenties earn its reputation. Sex advice became a topic of magazines; birth control was a talking point. For the first time sex memoirs appeared and advertising started to cash in on sexual imagery of women.

The new emphasis on sex and the pursuit of pleasure placed more demands on marriage. Individuals had only just written emotional fulfilment into the marital script, now they wanted sexual fulfilment too! Female writers claimed that a key ingredient to a successful marriage was sexual spice. As expectations increased so too did dissatisfaction, and divorce rates in the 1920s increased.

Just like today, social commentators seized on this, bandying around phrases such as 'the lost morals of youth', 'the disregard of marriage vows' and 'Is marriage bankrupt?' One book, *The Marriage Crisis* by sociologist Ernest Groves, claimed that the 'pursuit of the pleasure principle [sexual pleasure] was creating unrealistic expectations'. If Groves thought spousal expectations were high then, imagine what he would make of the demands we put on our partners today.

The same sociologist warned that the new craze for closeness required couples to place each other's needs above their families. This prompted other sociologists to rue that human behaviour was slowly changing from group to pair dynamics. Interesting that sociologists now talk of how human behaviour is slowly becoming focused on the individual.

This was a blessed generation. They were the first to personally choose their marital partners and they did so amid a glamorous backdrop of dance halls, champagne and cocaine. But they only got to live a few pages of their fairytale before practicality once more took over. The Great Depression of the 1930s brought everyone right back down to earth. Money became everyone's focus as wages dropped and jobs were cut.

Women were forced into the labour market, but rather than this being seen as empowering as it had the decade before, it was regarded as a humiliating necessity, as in the Victorian era. High-status positions were reserved for men so when a woman was forced to work, it was usually doing something laborious, like cleaning or seamstressing. Some American states brought in laws prohibiting women from certain professions. Three quarters of school systems wouldn't allow women teachers so that they could save the jobs for the men.[10]

The Second World War offered a brief respite from these sexually unjust employment laws. With men at war, women were needed in the workplace in all roles. Not as pretty secretaries but as mechanics, welders and carpenters, and they were paid the same rates as men. Women rejoiced in their new roles and revelled in a sense of purpose and achievement. But as soon as the war was over, they were chivvied back into their homemaker roles and men were reunited with their role as head of the household. Post-war governments in Western Europe and North America created tax systems and welfare programmes which strongly favoured male-breadwinner households. Magazines were rife with anti-feminist articles (many of them written by women!) accusing any woman who tried to continue her wartime job of 'castrating her husband'. Added to this, wages and standards of living increased across all classes after the Second World War, affording a positively golden standard of living compared to the hardships of the 1930s. But that didn't mean a return to the good times of dating and dancing as in the 1920s. After the horrors of war and a depression, there was a distinctly subdued mood and focus instead switched to the family. This is why marriage became the centre of society in the 1950s. Historians call it 'the golden age of marriage'. The male-breadwinning love-based coupling had been an ideal of the Victorian age but it was only now that the economic climate allowed the majority of the population to adopt it.

10 *The Changing Lives of American Women*, Steven D. McLaughlin. The University of North Carolina Press, USA, 1988

As historian Stephanie Coontz puts it: 'The 1950s were a culmination of ideals about marital satisfaction and male-female relationships that emerged in the nineteenth century and finally got realised in the twentieth.'

A united family front was the ultimate symbol of respectability. Securing a husband and starting a family was the gateway to adulthood for any young girl. People couldn't get hitched early enough. In most countries across Europe the percentage of 24-year-old men who were married in the early 1950s was twice as high as it had been 50 years earlier. By the 1960s 95 per cent of all people married at some point in their lives.[11]

Marriage was universal and viewed as permanent. Any lifestyle choice deviating from the marital norm was just short of shameful. One survey in 1957 found that four out of five people believed that anyone who preferred to remain single was 'sick, neurotic or immoral'.[12]

Literature shows bachelors being labelled 'immature', 'narcissistic' and even 'pathological'. Single women were described by psychiatrists of the day as 'sexually warped', 'lacking in the feminine instinct' and almost certainly suffering from a bad case of 'penis envy'. One leading family 'expert' of the 1950s said: 'Except for the sick, the badly crippled, the deformed, the emotionally warped, and the mentally defective, almost everyone could and should wed.'

Women invested in their family image with saccharine

---

11 *Marriage, a History: How Love Conquered Marriage*, Stephanie Coontz. Penguin USA, 2006.
12 *New Rules: Searching for Self-fulfillment in a World Turned Upside Down*, Daniel Yankelovich. Random House, 1981.

effort. If the phrase 'yummy mummy' was in use then, it would have been a fitting description for the typically conscientious housewife. I remember my grandma talking regularly about the importance of 'showing good face' – now I know what she was referring to. Husbands governed, wives baked cakes, couples stayed together, families did everything to maintain a sense of propriety. But no sooner had this fairytale ideal been achieved than it began to crumble.

Feelings of relief and gratitude from the hardships of the Second World War started to fade and focus once more edged towards individual goals and hedonistic pleasures. The booming economy, in need of more workers, started to tempt women back to employment – the very women who felt nostalgic about the wartime roles that they had reluctantly given up. The craze for labour-saving, household appliances like vacuum cleaners eased domestic chores. It was easy enough to live alone, perhaps? And then, in 1960, came the biggest influencer of all – the contraceptive pill.

Reliable contraception meant sex no longer came with life-changing consequences for women. The risk of pregnancy had been a barrier for recreational sex since, well, since man and woman figured out conception. Basically, women joined the party and premarital sex became the norm. Daring couples engaged in swinging and dreamt up games involving keys and fruit bowls (of more later). People began to discuss the possibility of open marriages and cohabitation before marriage became acceptable. Then in the 1970s monstrous inflation further weakened the male breadwinner model of marriage in sending even more women into the workforce.

By the 1980s, in the Western world the workforce was starting to resemble a level playing field. This introduced new hurdles into romantic relationships. Women no longer needed men's financial support so they started to look to them for more emotional support. Men complained that women demanded equal pay yet still expected them to pick up the tab. Women who didn't work became paranoid that they weren't pulling their financial weight and might be surplus to a man's needs. Those who did work became paranoid that they would neglect their families and disappoint their husbands. Worse still, there was a new strain of resentment bubbling under the surface over childcare. If both sexes were working full-time for similar wages, why should Mum always be the one to do bathtime? These sources of bickering would have been alien to other generations.

There was no precedent as to how these issues could be resolved and there still isn't. Marriage has slowly become less about necessity and more about choice. As a result we are still in a flux over what purpose it is supposed to serve.

* * *

The obvious debate raging in today's landscape of relationships is that of gay marriage. I smile whenever I see images of protesters carrying banners depicting couples in wedding gowns inside a red heart with the words 'Marriage = Man & Woman' because it had nothing to do with love until 200 years ago. Marriage, like language, laws, customs and Facebook privacy settings, constantly changes to reflect the temporaneous needs of the people, and commentators always fret about changes.

When we talk about losing touch with 'old fashioned values' or going back to 'traditional marriage', we are in fact referring to one short-lived period – the 1950s – which proved unsustainable anyway. It's no good squeezing round objects into square holes. We live in a world geared to convenience, autonomy, choice and unprecedented social networking. Basing our romantic relationships on an ideal that suited the social and economic climate six decades ago is anachronistic.

Perhaps a better approach to suit our times is to stop thinking of relationships as a necessity, as they have been throughout history, but as a luxury addition to our lives. Something to be enjoyed rather than to be leaned upon. We have never demanded so much from romantic relationships as we do today: we expect our long-term romantic partner to be our lover, our best friend, a devoted and disciplined parent, a sounding board on our career, an able DIY enthusiast, a bed fellow and a carer when we are sick. We want them to enjoy the company of the same sets of friends, to contribute to the household income and to take the garbage out. And on top of this we still expect romantic love to sizzle and for an arm in the middle of the night to cradle us.

I can't help thinking that in our agglomeration of what we want a relationship to serve, we've forgotten how to enjoy them. Perhaps it would be better to compartmentalise the benefits and joys of what our lovers can bring to our lives, rather than pigeon-holing them into some multi-purpose role spanning domesticity, career support and bedroom fireworks.

New couples are obsessed with destination despite there no longer being any pressing need for marriage. They move in together as soon as they're satisfied that neither of them has a criminal record or an incurable flesh-eating disease. Before they know it, they're attending family functions, they've given up reading novels in bed, they're not seeing the friends that their partner doesn't like and the giggling has given way to nagging about trimming toenails in front of the TV. We're so intent on 'moving things on' that we forget to enjoy the beautiful, fleeting stages of new love. The whole relationship becomes rooted in the minutiae of everyday tasks.

I'm not saying that we should do away with love and loyalty and instead engage in an endless flow of dalliances, never having to burden ourselves with emotional investment. In reality, civilised society would be unsustainable if the majority of us went through life like an 18–30s holiday. Work meetings would turn into orgies, men would have no one to iron their shirts and everyone would have the CSA child maintenance hotline saved to speed dial. We will continue to fall in love and to believe the feeling will last forever. But we should adopt a more grown-up approach to relationships. That means casting away the foolish fairytale that one person can answer all our needs. It means facing up to the fact that a life partner – should we choose to have one – fulfils only one corner of our emotional, romantic and sexual needs. And I shall prove this with science.

CHAPTER 5

Crazy for Love

Just because marriage was functional for all those thousands of years it didn't mean that humans were immune to love during those times. Although I don't think the full-time, committed girlfriend-boyfriend relationship will necessarily complement my busy lifestyle, that doesn't mean I'm going to stop falling in love either – far from it. Romantic love is the most highly charged human experience there is. It is probably the most written about, talked about, sung about, rhymed about, cried over, drunk over emotion we have. Except it isn't an emotion: it's a drive, like hunger.

Let me explain by putting it into the context of the simple crush. We all get them. The cute guy you see at the water cooler at work, the girl who lives at the end of your road, your personal trainer. You can't help it when you fancy someone, you just *do*. Your feelings creep up on you. You hardly notice them and then suddenly you're looking them up on Facebook and hoping to bump into them every time you leave the house. I'm particularly pathetic when I get a crush.

I had one recently, much to my annoyance because it stopped me from doing anything. I would catch my mind wandering at the most inappropriate moments to scenes where we would happen to meet. I'd lose concentration on what I was doing for just a second and suddenly we would be sitting on a bar stool after just arranging an excuse for an impromptu drink. Our knees would be touching and we'd be making subtle innuendo gestures. Then I would jolt myself back to my task in hand, which was probably trying to write 1,500 words by lunchtime.

For someone who doesn't care for a relationship, I am incurably weak when I have a crush. I allow it to take over my head. It lies in wait, monitoring my concentration and as soon as it shows so much as a twitch, the crush barges in, scattering tempting fantasies all over my consciousness. I only knew this particular one vaguely through a work project and I thought he was insightful, articulate and funny. But my seedling of a crush grew and within a few weeks I was convinced that he was funny, kind, intelligent and amazing in bed. He could well have been a total idiot and gay for all I knew, but for whatever mystical reason – his turn of phrase, his gestures, whatever – he had triggered a response in me that was now usurping all my attention.

What I now know is that my 'romantic love system' had been triggered. Dr Helen Fisher is an anthropologist who has dedicated her whole career to studying the chemical and anatomical explanations of love. She has spent decades examining brain scans of honeymoon couples, long-term couples, randy lovers and more.

I first interviewed Dr Fisher several years ago for a newspaper and her theory resonated with me more than any other expert, sexpert, academic or scientist that I have ever interviewed. The science of attraction. Who wouldn't be fascinated in that? For weeks afterwards, I rattled it off to anyone who would listen. Romantic love, Dr Fisher explained, is one of three different drives that make up the brain's system for attraction: we have a sex drive, a drive for romantic love and a drive for attachment.

No prizes for guessing what the sex drive is responsible for. It's linked to the hormone testosterone and its evolutionary purpose for our prehistoric ancestors was to encourage us to copulate and – thank goodness – secure the continuation of the human race.

The drive for romantic love is less talked about but experienced much more strongly. It is linked with the feel-good chemicals dopamine and norepinephrine. Its evolutionary purpose was to motivate us to woo and win a particular partner and to make us enamoured enough to start building a family with them. You see, back in the days of caveman and cavewoman, babies would not have fared well had they been born to a single female. Mothers needed a mate to protect them from prey (and give her his hunted meat when she was trying to stop the baby crying). The tender cavemen and women who fell in love produced offspring more likely to survive. And so, over centuries those brain networks for falling in romantic love were passed down until they became an inherent part of being human.

Romantic love is by its very nature a bit trippy. It makes us obsessed and immune to any of our love object's faults. Because of that it wouldn't make evolutionary sense for caveman and cavewoman to remain in a state of romantic love forever. They'd never get round to any cavehold chores or finding food. So nature gave us a drive for attachment.

Attachment is linked to the hormone oxytocin – known as

the 'cuddle hormone' because it gets released through human touch, or any affectionate touch. Animals feel it too. The reason your dog loves resting his head on your stomach? It's getting a hit of oxytocin from the body contact. This is why we love our backs being stroked so much. We also release oxytocin when we feel long-term familiarity, trust and companionship for someone. Our drive for attachment evolved to make caveman and cavewoman stay together even after the rollercoaster of romantic love had calmed down.

Unlike most mammals, humans walk on two legs. This meant our ancestors had to carry babies in their arms rather than their mouths, or on their backs over dangerous ground and so they were more prey to hunters. 'If you had to carry something the size of a bowling ball around with you, you would find a mate pretty fast!' notes Dr Fisher. 'It was essentially our physical limitations that caused our reliance on sexual partners. Our brains evolved a system for love and feelings of deep attachment to reflect the demands of our environment.'

These drives evolved something like four million years ago but the drive for romantic love is the strongest of them all, even stronger than our sex drive. 'If you are sexually attracted to someone and they turn down your sexual offers, you don't go killing yourself. But if you are romantically attracted to them, rejection is far more severe,' explains Dr Fisher. 'People stalk over romantic love; they can even kill over romantic love.' This all made sense to me. Not that I've ever stalked or killed anyone I've had the hots for, but it does explain why I can't get any work done.

'When the romantic love system is triggered, we lose control. The person you desire becomes the centre of your world. You become obsessive, you get lots of energy, you become elated when you see them, you begin to crave them and you become highly motivated to win them. You are likely to do anything for them, even die for them. The attachment drive is much less fervent. When you are attached to someone you trust them deeply and you miss that person when you are not with them. But you're rational.'

Finally I felt like I could make sense of love. This ardent feeling that we call courtly love, or lust or passion, chemistry, a crush or a magic spark is all explicable by dopamine. The tummy somersaults, the racing heart rate, the food of writers and philosophers from Shakespeare to Plato is a drive controlled by a hormone that doesn't sound too dissimilar to a Disney character.

All my past crushes and unsuitable love affairs now felt legitimate. Any embarrassment over going wobbly at the knees because I've fancied an elusive figure; any of those 'what-was-I-thinking?' moments over expensive long-haul flights to visit an overseas lover who didn't even speak my language; all those expensive cab rides across London in the middle of the night in my younger days to a party where I thought a certain guy might be. All those things were perfectly normal reactions within my romantic love system.

This makes attraction three-dimensional. There is sexual attraction – obviously. There is social attraction – when you get on with someone and enjoy their company. But there is also a third, crucial but overlooked dimension: romantic attraction. This is the elusive 'spark'. That's why you can find someone physically attractive and perfectly agreeable too. They are probably charming, clever and reliable but you just don't feel the magic. So, the next time my friends asked why I didn't 'give him a chance', I decided I would simply reply, 'Oh, I'm just not feeling any dopamine.'

I have an acquaintance who had a raging crush on a colleague at the office where she worked as an IT consultant. She really thought there was something there. They'd had coffees and lunches together and as her crush grew, despite him being engaged, she started to think of ways that she could increase her contact with him or things she could do that would attract his attention. He was into climbing and used a local climbing wall. So what did she do? She joined too.

It worked to an extent. She now had an excuse to make conversation with him – they'd turn up to work with all their ropes and clips and helmets and have a little chuckle about it. Six months – and no dates – later, she was climbing up some rocks in Wales and had a dreadful accident and broke several limbs and her back. She spent more than a year in hospital and lost her hair through the shock.

A whole 18 months after her accident, still learning to walk again, she returned to work and had to face the colleague who had inspired her to go climbing in the first place. While she had been in hospital, he had got married!

Weeks after returning to work, the team was invited to her boss's home for a work function and she was forced to greet his beautiful, cheerful wife while she was still walking with a frame. They had a dream four-bedroom home. 'I looked around and thought I wouldn't want this and him anyway. He's actually quite a boring guy. I can't start to think that my accident was because of him because I'd go crazy if I thought that, but I do wish I could have pressed the off button when I felt my feelings for him grow,' she reflected.

But the thing with romantic love is there is no off button. Dr Helen Fisher says it is typical to become 'highly motivated' to win our infatuate. My friend certainly had high motivations to win her colleague and what a brutal price she paid. But she was no different and no more obsessive than any of us.

My previous 'high motivations' to attract the attentions of certain men have included buying outfits I couldn't afford, going on a camping holiday when I hate camping, growing my hair and, when I was 18, changing my walking route to my part-time job in a sandwich shop, adding a whole 15 minutes to my journey in the hope that he'd spot me walking along the bypass as he drove to work. Quite what I thought would happen if he did see me walking on the bypass is beyond me.

'Obsession,' states Dr Fisher, 'is the essential component of romantic love. Being in love means being obsessed.' And how does she know this? Because she put 17 people who had either been rejected or had strong feelings for someone they couldn't have into a brain scanner. The patterns from the neuroimaging turned out to be exactly the same as someone with a crack cocaine addiction.

The areas of the brain for cravings and addiction were raging with activity. 'I looked at the data and I thought these are drives!' Dr Fisher exclaimed. 'Not emotions. If you are angry with someone you can get over it in the afternoon – because it is an emotion. But if you are hungry, or thirsty, or you are craving your addicted substance, you remain thirsty or hungry, or craving your addiction, until you get what you need. These three systems – sex, romantic love and attachment – are no different.'

But Dr Helen Fisher wasn't the first to look into our desirous nature, she was just the first to do so with technology. In the 1970s psychologist Dorothy Tennov wrote a whopper of a book called *Love and Limerence*. 'Limerence' was a word she came up with to describe the 'involuntary state of mind which results from romantic attraction and leads to an overwhelming, obsessive need to have your feelings reciprocated'. She decided the concept needed a name after interviewing her students about their feelings of love and attraction and finding that most had quite drastic stories to tell of the effects of limerence. Some missed whole terms of lessons; others described having intrusive thoughts. Such an emotionally charged state deserved its own term, she believed. 'Love' didn't really do it justice and it was obviously stronger than finding a girl in a short skirt sexy.

* * *

It says something about the complexity of romantic attraction when you need yet another word to describe it. Especially if you consider the rich lexicon we already have: infatuation, lust, a crush, puppy love, new love, obsessive love, romantic love. Did we really need limerence? Tennov thought we did.

It also says something when romantic love and limerence form the central theme of the most well known stories in literature and legend. Romantic longings have spurred writers and artists to create their greatest masterpieces. Love has been the backbone of fiction, plays, songs, poems, letters, tragedies, sit-coms, films, fairytales, sages, myths and legends throughout the ages.

The world's alleged first novel, *The Tale of Genji*, written in Japan in the early eleventh century, was a love story telling of a handsome prince's frustration as he continually fell in love with forbidden women. Almost every piece of classic literature ever since has followed the same theme. *Gone with the Wind*, *Jane Eyre*, *Pride and Prejudice*, *The Scarlet Pimpernel* and *Wuthering Heights* are all about elusive love. Or there are those that concentrate on the physical yearnings of romantic love: *The Scarlet Letter*, *Madame Bovary*, *The Canterbury Tales*, *Lady Chatterley's Lover* and *Anna Karenina*.

As for poets, they simply gorge on the stuff. The *Amarushataka* (One Hundred Poems of Amaru), written in Sanskrit in around the eighth century is considered one of the highest-ranking collections of lyrical poetry. There is verse after verse on erotic love, estrangement, longing, rapprochement, courting, consummation, betrayal, feminine forms and masculine ego.

Anthologies of love letters from the likes of Ernest Hemingway, Elizabeth Barrett Browning, Jack London, Dylan Thomas, Franz Kafka, George Sand, George Bernard Shaw, Oscar Wilde, Katherine Mansfield and Lewis Carroll are so appealing to us because they overspill with passionate prose for absent lovers.

Love in literature is nearly always obsessive. *The Great Gatsby*, which has been made into a film many times over, is the story of the obsessive love of Jay Gatsby for his old flame Daisy Buchanan. Gatsby put his entire life on hold, believing that she would one day leave her husband and they would be reunited. He bought a mansion on the opposite side of Long Island Bay from where Daisy lived so 'he could be near her'. Every weekend for years he hosted great elaborate parties and invited all of New York's high society in the hope that one day, Daisy would show up: she didn't.

Opera is a parody of romantic love, its staple storyline featuring a hero tormented by rejection. In *The Phantom of the Opera*, the opera ghost (who is really just a sad, deformed, unattractive man) falls obsessively in love with the lead singer of the opera and is forced to watch her fall in love with someone else. He can't bear it and so he kidnaps her. Similarly, in *Notre Dame de Paris* the bell ringer Quasimodo is tortured by his love for the gypsy girl Esmeralda and he too kidnaps her, on the orders of his adopted father. In *The Divine Comedy*, the protégé Dante has been in love with the character Beatrice since he was nine, even though he's only met her twice.

But although it's OK to be affected by obsessive romantic love in literature, if we owned up to such emotions in the real world we'd probably find ourselves with a restraining order. The only person you can admit to being enamoured with is a proper boyfriend or girlfriend or fiancé or spouse. You have to know them really well or else it isn't love. I remember teenage magazines telling me I couldn't be 'in love' unless I knew a man's faults as well as his good points. I've heard friends say you can't really know a person properly unless you've lived with them. And I've read agony aunts sneering at the idea of 'love at first sight' – love is much deeper, they concede smugly. But Hemingway, Shakespeare, Goethe and the Brontë sisters didn't think so.

One of Dr Helen Fisher's studies found that a quarter of people say they've experienced love at first sight. 'All it takes is for someone to trigger the dopamine system in your brain and for you to be open to falling in love,' she explained. 'If someone walks into a supermarket, they are smiling, they are wearing a T-shirt with your favourite sports team and they are humming a song you relate to, that can be enough to trigger it. It's most often triggered at times of change. When people move to another country, get a new job, inherit a lot of money or lose a lot of money, it creates novelty and with that you feel more susceptible to falling in love. It isn't surprising that people fall in romantic love during warfare. As horrible as it is, the adrenalin is rushing, you are not with your usual friends. The brain is enlivened and your dopamine systems are easily triggered.'

The philosopher Francis Bacon went so far as to say that new giddy love was a curse. In his classic essay 'Of Love' in the sixteenth century he warned men that they 'ought to beware of this passion, which loseth not only other things, but itself!' and lambasted love as something that 'ruined good men'. He said that love played a great role on the stage but in real life it was 'more troublesome' and could lead a man to ignore his work, concluding 'it is impossible to love, and to be wise'.

The ancient Greeks thought love was a type of insanity. Medieval philosophers in France came to the same conclusion, defining it as a 'derangement of the mind' that could be cured only by sex.[13] In the eighteenth century and closer to home, *The Treasury of Encyclopedia Britannica* (like Wikipedia before the Internet) included an entry for 'love in medicine'. It listed a range of symptoms resulting from this 'passion as a disease', which included hollow eyes, irregular pulse, deep sighs, loss of appetite, melancholy, and, it could result in madness or even death!

Today romantic love is often dismissed as 'just lust', 'just a fling' or 'puppy love'. Perhaps the disapproval and the unwillingness to take it seriously occur because society only gives moral recognition to enduring love. New boyfriends

---

[13] *Marriage, a History: How Love Conquered Marriage*, Stephanie Coontz. Penguin USA, 2006

never merit a 'plus one' on a wedding invite. Unrequited love is never considered as heartbreaking as a 'proper' break up. Hell, Romeo killed himself for a girl he'd spent one night with! But that's OK because he was Romeo.

Here's the irony. What all my married friends declare as 'proper love' isn't romantic love. It's actually 'attachment' and concerns a whole different group of brain chemicals (some scientists define it as 'companionate love'). This distinction has been referenced variously by many scholars over many years. For example, in the1800s the philosopher Søren Kierkegaard, who wrote extensively about passion, proposed that erotic love was addictive and put the mind in an altered state. He said that erotic love leads us to believe it will be forever, but it is never forever. And that's why we should love our neighbours because affectionate love is more reliable.

In one of his books, *Diary of a Seducer*, which Kierkegaard wrote under a pseudonym, he advised that 'no love affair should last more than half a year at most'. To him the whole point of romantic love or erotic love, or whatever phrase you wish to use, was the chase. 'Once resistance is gone love is only weakness and habit,' he wrote. Which is the same thing as saying once you've got your mitts on the person you want, you'll both start burping and bickering, and you'll want to chase someone else.

Centuries before Kierkegaard, a more famous name illustrated the incompatibility of romantic love and longevity: William Shakespeare. Many of his plays convey the message that marriage and romance are not in tune with each other. In *Measure for Measure*, for example, the heroine Isabella needs love, and that's exactly why she considers rejecting marriage with the Duke. All he wants, you see, is an heir. But she wants more. He portrays a similarly cynical view of romantic marriage in *Twelfth Night* and *Hamlet*.

And while I'm on the subject, the ancient Greeks distinguished between four types of love: *Eros* for the passionate stuff which by default comes with physical desire and longing; *Agape*, the deep unconditional love for a long-term partner or family member associated with contentment and security; *Philia*, a brotherly, virtuous love felt for friends or a community and associated with loyalty and respect, and finally, *Storge*, which is merely a soft affection – a fondness through familiarity.

The Greeks gave great intellectual consideration to defining love. In *Symposium* the great philosopher Plato envisaged what all his most learned friends would say about it. He wrote a fictionalised account of an elite dinner party hosted in the winter of 416 BC, to which the finest intellectuals of Athens were invited to discuss love. Plato imagined what each character, including Socrates (with whom he was well acquainted in real life) would say.

Bear in mind that Symposiums were not unlike dinner parties of today. The guests would often get blind drunk and embellish stuff, so their theories were imaginative to say the least. Aristophanes, for instance, attempted to explain why people in love say they feel 'whole'. In primal times, he told the dinner table, people had double bodies with two heads and two sets of limbs. The creatures were very powerful, but cheeky by the sounds of it, because they tried to scale the heights of heaven and take over the gods. I suppose one would call it a mythological coup.

Zeus, the father of all the gods, fought back and in his anger he chopped them in half – separating them into two beings. He then commanded his son Apollo, the god of medicine and healing, to turn their faces around and stitch them up from the navel but not to heal the navel so that Man would always be reminded of this event. Ever since, people have been running around saying they are looking for their 'other half'.

Socrates offered up another gem of a theory. At a wild birthday party hosted by the God Aphrodite, Resource, the son of Invention, got drunk and crashed out to sleep in the garden. Poverty crept up on Resource and slept with him, hoping to relieve her lack of resources by having a child with him. Love was the child that Poverty conceived by Resource. So, Socrates concluded, as the child of Resource and Poverty, love will always be poor, but very tough. He will sleep outdoors, like his mother, always in a state of need, but like his father, he can scheme to get whatever he wants.

* * *

Thankfully, we now have the benefits of science over the lucid imaginations of drunken Greek philosophers and bereft writers to explain what love is. We have archaeological tools, DNA testing, hormone detectors, brain scan imagery and more to understand the biological and chemical reactions in our bodies. I wonder how Plato's dinner guests would have reacted had Dr Helen Fisher been at the Symposium and talked about surges of dopamine and norepinephrine and comparing love to crack addiction? But it looks pretty bleak for new couples hopeful their love will last forever. Must that lovely passionate, fuzzy, topsy-turvy tummy feeling of romantic love always be short-lived? Is it always doomed to fade and then we'll adopt boring old feelings of attachment as we become more familiar with each other?

Some anthropologists say that the natural lifespan of romantic love is around seven years because that's how long it would take to raise a brood of children to relative independence. We are hardwired for our romantic desires to redirect after this time because it serves our species well if we mix up the gene pool up a bit. Scientific evidence you might say for the seven-year itch.

Some studies show that levels of vasopressin (the aggression hormone) are higher in couples who have been together longer, indicating that we become more frustrated with each other as time goes on.[14] Many tribal cultures openly observe this time limit on romantic love. In a traditional Canela marriage ceremony in Brazil the bride and groom lie on the floor together while their uncles tell them to stay together until their eldest child has grown up and in the meantime not to get jealous of each other's lovers.[15]

There's even more bad news for romantics, I'm afraid. Even the long-term, companionate love can also decline. Psychology professor Elaine Hatfield carried out a study in 1981 that found that the affectionate emotions associated with long-term commitment sometimes decline at the same rate as romantic love. There are exceptions to the rule. Dr Helen Fisher told me some of her experiments on long-term couples showed that their romantic love systems were still active even after 40 years and they were still emitting brainwaves that resembled addiction. 'But it is rare,' she admitted.

All this makes me think that while there is still a place for

---

14 *No More Silly Love Songs: A Realist's Guide to Romance*, Anouchka Grose. Portobello Books, London, 2011
15 *Mother Nature: Maternal Instincts and How They Shape the Human Species*, Sarah Blaffer Hrdy. Ballantine Books, 2000

long-term, deep, robust relationships for those who want them, that model will always be challenged by the more forceful drive for fervent, passionate, new romantic love. Never has the force been so strong as it is today. The Internet guarantees us anonymity for affairs, a faster paced life means we become bored more easily, better health allows us to live longer and stay sexually active later, modern domestic appliances and services permit us to live alone, giving us leverage to walk away from a stale relationship.

We never used to expect romantic love to last forever, which is why we kept it outside of marriage. Ever since we aspired to marry the one we love, the central challenge has been how to prevent love going stale amid the prosaic realities of sharing a roof, a social life and holidays. Much as I am loath to admit it, the scientific evidence proves that the stability of long-term attachment and the excitement of romantic love are two different forces. The conventional fairytale marriage doesn't look so strong wavering in between the two.

CHAPTER 6

Not Tonight, Darling –
I'm Asexual

Aside from utter denial of reality, the other illuminating thing about love and limerence is sex. When someone gets our dopamine going, we want to rip his pants off! At least most of us do. Asexuals don't. As the name suggests, Asexuality is a permanent, endemic lack of sexuality. That doesn't just mean a low libido. It doesn't refer to bored couples or exhausted mothers who just can't be bothered any more, it refers to those who have never had a libido at all.

But here's the interesting thing – even though asexuals don't experience sexual attraction, they still fancy people. The ones I spoke to described attraction as something much stronger than platonic friendship but totally independent of sexual longing.

I met Estelle, a 25-year-old PhD history student at York University. She'd been with her asexual boyfriend for two years. They've never had sex and never intend to. She came to meet me alone. Her boyfriend was too busy, or rather too shy, she later admitted. They met through an asexual support group called AVEN (The Asexual Visibility and Education Network). A petite and pretty energetic girl, Estelle had red hair, freckled skin and not a jot of make-up.

'I am so in love with my boyfriend, I can't describe how much I love him!' Estelle chirped, once we started talking about her relationship. 'We share lots of physical intimacy. We kiss and cuddle up in bed – we can't keep our hands off each other sometimes! So it's certainly not platonic love but it's not sexual either. I've felt love for my friends but the love for them isn't romantic. What I have for my boyfriend is *very* different to that.'

'Have you always had asexual relationships?' I asked.

'If only! This is my first. I wish I'd known before that there were other people like me who were happy not to have sex. I got into my first relationship when I was 19 and it lasted two and a half years. At the time I felt embarrassed that I'd never had a relationship. Society pressures you to be in one and sex is an expected part of that. I wasn't repulsed by sex but I was uncomfortable with it and I didn't know why. I liked being in a relationship but I felt no interest in having sex. I felt like I had to do it to keep the relationship going; that created a conflict inside me. Then I started to resent sex.

'After we split, the opportunity for a new relationship soon arose. I was attracted to him and wanted to be with him but when we had a couple of dates and I started to pick up that he wanted sex, the conflict came back. It felt like I had to do it to continue the relationship. But I felt so uncomfortable about it, not excited by it at all, even puzzled why people would want to do it. Sex seems so uncivilised to me. When I'm attracted to someone, I feel the same as anyone else. I feel a longing to be with them and I want to touch them but the sexual aspect has never been part of that longing.

'I forced myself to have sex with him a few times but I think he picked up that I wasn't into it and we fizzled out. For the next two years I struggled with sexual relationships. I had the whole flirtatious thing going on with a few guys, but then I would stop dead and think, "Oh God, I'm going to have to have sex!" That would destroy it for me and I'd stop flirting. I just wasn't prepared to put myself through it, so I stayed out of a relationship for two years.

'One day the word asexual came up in a conversation and a light bulb went on. It felt like I had found out who I was; I had a whole new pathway to follow. I felt liberated. Society constantly tells you that you need a partner and you should be having sex with that partner but when I discovered that I was part of another group, it was like the rules of society didn't apply to me anymore.'

For Estelle romantic love is independent of sexual desire. Actually it probably is for all of us but because sexual feelings are inextricably linked to romantic feelings the two usually overlap. Romantic attraction often becomes sexual attraction and vice versa. There have been many times when I've been attracted to a man solely because of what he does to me intellectually or because he makes me laugh. I may not have found him physically attractive at first but over time that romantic spark evolves into physical attraction.

The term sapiosexual is a recently coined buzzword I hear a lot of women use to indicate that they are sexually attracted to someone's intellect. I can recall many men I've been drawn to but not wanted to jump into bed with immediately. Sometimes it's confused me. But it's those initial feelings of attraction – romantic attraction – that set the foundations for sexual passion to grow.

* * *

Key to the self-identify of asexuals is the concept of romantic orientation. It relates to which sex they are romantically attracted. Just as we can be homosexual or heterosexual, we can also be homoromantic or heteroromantic. Most people are sexually attracted to the same sex that they are romantically attracted to. So you get the physical desire to tear their clothes off, along with the romantic desire to take a long walk with them and gaze into their eyes.

But not always: sometimes there's a clash. A gay man for instance may be homosexual with a full and flavourful sex life with other men. But he could also be heteroromantic if he is attracted to women in a romantic way. Perhaps he has a special female friend whom he adores and looks out for and shares a bed with but has no desire to make love to. Or a straight woman could be heterosexual, fancying guys and sleeping with them just like her straight friends, but she could also be homoromantic and crave an intimate, close relationship – minus the sex – with another woman.

Asexuals are of course neither homosexual nor heterosexual because they have no sexual orientation. But they do have a romantic one. (There is one current area of research into the idea of a-romanticism – those who have no romantic attraction at all. This disturbs me because I imagine someone who has never daydreamed about anyone or never stared at their phone willing it to flash up with a certain person's number is nothing short of sociopathic.)

Estelle and her boyfriend were heteroromantic. The next

couple I met, Heather and Trisha, identified as homoromantic. At 38 and 40, they had been together for five years. When they first got in touch with me they described themselves as 'a madly in love couple who are total monogamists'.

'What do you mean by monogamists?' I asked when we met. 'If you don't have sex with anyone, how could you ever be unfaithful?'

'What monogamy means to me is that sometimes we can come across other women and think, yes, there's romantic compatibility here, but we wouldn't try to pursue it,' said Heather, a sales director. She had long dark-blonde high-lighted hair tied in a tight ponytail and was wearing a black skirt suit and big chunky heels.

'We might come across people that appeal to us as friends, but who we don't necessarily feel romantically compatible with,' added Trisha. The two women looked similar – Trisha had darker hair but their styles and their business dress sense were the same. 'And that's fine to start a friendship. But a romantic relationship would be very different to starting a friendship with someone. It would be very clear that it was more than friendship.'

'We have lots of strong friendships with men and women,' continued Heather. 'But it's different somehow to romantic feelings. I don't want to touch those friends but me and Heather love touch and affection.' They looked at each other and gave a knowing smile. Often they touched each other's shoulders or gave each other's hands a squeeze throughout the whole interview.

'Have either of you ever had sex with anyone before you knew you were asexual?' I asked.

'I haven't,' stated Heather. 'But I'm rare. What you'll find with most asexuals is that before they identify as asexual they succumb to the pressure to fit in and then have an epiphany when they discover that asexuality exists. I never understood the concept of sexual attraction. When I was young, I thought sex was something people did if they wanted children. As I grew up, I started to learn that sex is something you do with someone you love, but I thought it was quite disgusting. At age 11 or 12 when friends at school were learning about the facts of life and sharing what they knew in the playground, I remember thinking, "How gross!" I never thought it would apply to me. Then a few years later when friends began pairing off with boys at school that was evidence that there is this thing called sexual attraction, which for most people follows romantic love.

'Once that clicked, I kept waiting, assuming that I too would feel sexual attraction sometime. I got together with a boy and kept thinking the feeling would develop once the relationship got going, but that just wasn't true.'

'Did he want sex?'

'*Did* he! He kept bringing it up all the time. But my feeling was primarily disgust. He didn't pressure me; he said the emotional part was more important. But there came a point where he became frustrated and the relationship ended. Even so, I still kept thinking I was going to experience this thing called sexual attraction with someone else but it never came. When I was about 20, I still hadn't had sex. I worried that I had some mental illness! I became depressed – I felt ashamed that I didn't want sex. Then one day I googled "Does everyone want sex?" and articles on asexuality came up and everything clicked. When I read it, I cried over my keyboard.'

Trisha touched and squeezed Heather's hand again, a little nudge of acknowledgement that she'd just disclosed something touchingly personal. 'I wasn't as sure of myself as Heather,' Trisha picked up. 'I let boyfriends persuade me into having sex. I didn't know about asexuality until after university. As soon as I heard the word I knew that was what I was. Even now I'm nervous about telling people I'm asexual. The immediate reactions are, "You're repressed, you're gay, you're frigid or you haven't met the right person". Even my parents said, "Are you sure you aren't gay?" when I came out as asexual. There is more anxiety among asexuals about coming out than there is among gay people.'

* * *

Estelle and her boyfriend and Heather and Trisha were lucky. They had their 'light bulb moments' early enough to take action and find a relationship model to suit them. Both couples met through AVEN. To find it, all they had to do was type words into Google and doors opened to help them find like-minded people. There are also asexual dating websites catering for both asexual people or those who've opted for celibacy for various reasons. Platonicpartners.co.uk is the fastest growing of these. Many of its members are older and don't consider sex an important part of companionship. Others have medical conditions, injuries or are impotent. Whatever their reasons, they still want a loving and fulfilling partnership. Thanks to the miracle of the Internet, they have an immediate solution to a life-long loveless struggle. But such niche communities weren't accessible before the digital age and so there are many asexuals who grew up struggling to understand their condition and never allowing themselves to love, simply because they couldn't bear the thought of sex.

Tim, a maths professor at a prestigious university is one such person. He grew up long before the Internet could help him out. At 52, he had never, ever experienced a love affair – not even a brief one – although this is something he has craved his whole life.

He greeted me with a warm handshake. His brown curly hair looked like it was a few weeks past its due date for a cut. Wearing dark denim jeans, a white shirt and a green corduroy jacket, he had a big smile, big glasses and a kind face. He didn't look like an award-winning internationally acclaimed maths genius at all. Nor did he look like a virgin. But he was both of those.

He led me into his office, a tiny room stacked with boxes overspilling with books. It was just as you would imagine an academic's room to be. He shared it with three others but this afternoon it was just the two of us. He shuffled around nervously and offered me a vending machine coffee. Once we'd broken the ice by talking about his latest research paper and my distant memories of A-level maths calculus, I asked when he first identified himself as being asexual.

'As far back as I can remember, I never wanted sex but I just didn't have a word for it,' he explained. He seemed to relax now that he sensed the interview proper was under-way, perhaps more comfortable talking about a set topic than small talk with a stranger. Well spoken, he told me he came from a military family and had been educated at public school.

'At any point in my life if you'd asked if I had experienced sexual attraction, I would have said no. Growing up, I observed my peers experiencing sexual attraction so I knew I was different in some way. My friends would say things like, "Isn't she hot?" or "Wouldn't you want to see her in her underwear?" But I couldn't relate to it. People would shove an explicit picture of a girl in front of me and I would think, "I don't know what the fuss is about."

'It didn't worry me because it didn't cause me discomfort. Not fitting in wasn't pleasant but I was happy – I had a nice life,' he shrugged, before adding, 'Saying that, there was pressure at school. Being sexually attracted to women is an expectation for a guy, especially in all-male situations and I went to an all-male school. We'd go out of our way not to "act like a gay". But if you're not interested in women of course the natural assumption is that you're gay. So I'd find myself doing more macho things to make up for it. I'd play lots of sport and make crude jokes with men. I disguised it up until my 30s, then it became glaringly obvious that I'd never had a girlfriend so the gay suspicions came back.'

'Do you tell them you're asexual now?' I asked.

'I don't go shouting it from rooftops but if it comes up, I openly use the term asexual. When I do, even as an adult the dominant response is, "You've not met the right person". The funniest response was, "Are you saving yourself for marriage?" Saving myself? I'm 52! The idea that people might never get into sex isn't within people's comprehension. It's these sorts of reactions that drive many asexuals into a relationship to try to overcome it. That causes all sorts of inner conflict. I'm not saying that it's wrong for asexuals to have a relationship with a sexual person but it's important for both sides to understand the other's needs and desires – it's a disaster if you don't tell your partner your hang-ups about sex. I know some asexuals who have sex with their partner because they love them and they want to make them happy and it's something they do as an act of love. Some asexuals have had sex in order to have children – they know it's something they must do. But for me the very idea of sex repulses me. Having sex would be a really big deal – it's not an option to even consider.'

Tim sighed and continued, 'I know that sex is an important part of what makes people feel good about themselves and I wouldn't want to be with a woman who kept thinking there was something wrong with her because I didn't desire her. I do crave a special one-on-one bond, I really do. But I resigned myself to the idea that I'd never have a relationship a very long time ago. I have close friendships and they suffice.'

I told Tim about Estelle and her boyfriend, and Heather and Trisha, and how they had found wonderful asexual partners and that perhaps he too could find all those things he yearned for – cuddling and intimacy and physical touch but without the sex.

'I've heard of AVEN and platonic dating sites,' he said. 'Maybe if I had something like that when I was younger, I would have used them. It would be hard to adapt now – I've set myself up for surviving alone. A lot of people think I'm weird. Society is geared towards couples and families and most people's aim in life is to find a partner. People can't comprehend that anything else could be the case.'

I ceased delving any deeper for I could sense that I'd stirred buried feelings. The warm smile that he greeted me with was replaced with a defeatist half-smile. How sad, I thought, that we are so conditioned to view sex and love as inextricably bound that Tim has been forced to exclude himself from both in order to avoid one.

And Tim was not alone in being forced into a solo life. Peter, a 32-year-old ceramic sculptor, had also lived a loveless life. Unlike Tim, he had tried and endured sex in an attempt to find love. Peter didn't want to meet me so we spoke over Skype: 'I have fallen in love with people so many times in my head but 100 per cent of the time it has been unrequited.' He was sitting in his studio but his screen was dark and I could only make out his silhouette and an obscured view of his face. It looked as if he was surrounded by papers, photos, pens, clay-like moulds and paintpots. He looked dishevelled but not unattractive. His style of speaking was formal, calm and articulate to the point of being scripted.

'Around puberty I noticed that I didn't seem to find girls quite as fascinating as other people my age did. I thought I could be gay because I found some people of my own gender emotionally interesting and alluring, but not sexually arousing. At the time I was tempted by sex and thought maybe if I was in a certain situation it would all click into place and I'd feel sexual, but it didn't.

'I had a number of attempts with both men and women over a number of years but with no results,' he sighed, relaxing a little now. 'I always liked the physical intimacy, I liked the hugging and affection but when it got to the interfering of bits and pieces – ugh! I didn't want to go near them, if I'm totally honest!' But Peter did because he thought that's what was expected of him. Unaroused by women he experimented with men, but still had no reaction other than, as he put it, 'the sort of screwy-up face you pull if you have to put your hand down a plughole to unblock all the hair.'

'I'd like to have loved and built up a life with many of the people that I had sexual encounters with,' he continued in his formal, unaffected tone. 'From what I read and hear, it seems many long-term marriages end up being sexless anyway. But it seems you need the sex and lust in the beginning to cement that special bond. I think once the person you are having sex with has become sufficiently emotionally close then the relationship evolves into something else and it doesn't matter if the sex stops, but carnal knowledge seems to be the cement that keeps you together.'

I liked his frankness. We all know it, but few of us accept it. There is no shortage of articles and jokes about spouses who complain that their sex life is non-existent and they have become like friends or siblings. Perhaps instead of finding a waning sex life frustrating, we should accept it. Historically, this is also why marriages must be consummated. Sex is what seals the relationship, but once sealed it's left to mature into whatever you make it, sexual or not.

As gay marriage was being hotly contested among the Commons and the Lords in 2013, one of the difficulties faced by civil servants in setting out the proposals for gay marriage was the question of what constitutes consummation. So awkward were the discussions about this that it was decided that judges could decide on a case-by-case basis. They may not have wanted to talk about sex acts during a parliamentary debate but it was clear that some sort of consummation would be needed to legitimise a life partnership.

Talking of sex acts, I had to ask Peter something you will no doubt also be wondering: 'Forgive me for asking, but without a sex drive do you still have the need to relieve yourself?' Very delicately put.

'Yes, I do,' he replied, unphased. 'Sex drive and sex orientation are different things. It is possible to lack sexual orientation but still have an urge that needs to be dealt with. I am capable of becoming aroused and having orgasms but what leads me to be aroused is purely physiological. The method I use to relieve those urges doesn't involve visualising anyone else or anything else. A good analogy would be, put a heterosexual man on a desert island where there are only men. He would still have urges but he wouldn't necessarily fantasise about those men.'

Peter was so clinical in his analogies it sounded like he could have been reading from a textbook. I wondered if that came from a life-long lack of romance and intimacy. If I stay single forever, will I one day become this dispassionate? If I don't have anyone to have a private giggle with, will my views also start to sound so monochrome?

* * *

The fear of 'coming out' and the shame of not fitting in is a common thread among all of the asexual people described above. Many of their stories echoed those of gay friends who've admitted that they too tried to force themselves into heterosexual relationships before they had the maturity and self-confidence to identify with their minority sexual orientation.

The parallels between homosexuality and asexuality don't stop there, though. Homosexuality wasn't officially declassified as a mental health disorder until shockingly late – 1973. That was when it was taken off the Diagnostic and Statistical Manual of Mental Disorders (DSM), which was established by the American Psychiatric Association and dubbed the 'mental health bible' because it lists and describes all the recognised psychiatric conditions. The World Health Organisation didn't remove it from its list of psychiatric disorders until even later – 1977. Gay sexual activity was illegal in the UK until 1967 and is still illegal in more than 70 countries.

The Gay Rights Movement started to battle for equality back in the 1970s. Most of the hard work has been done and, on the whole, homosexuality is now accepted as a normal variation of sexuality in Europe and the English-speaking world. Any remaining stigma is mostly due to religious protests. But there has been little groundwork laid to get asexuals fully integrated into society. Here's some shocking evidence as to how bigoted we are to sexless relationships. More than four decades after homosexuality was removed from the DSM, asexuality is still hidden in there.

The DSM recognises something it calls Hypoactive Sexual Desire Disorder (HSDD) or Sexual Aversion Disorder. It's characterised as a lack of sexual desire or sexual fantasies. But – and there's a *big* but – for it to be regarded as a disorder, the sufferer must actually report feeling distressed about it. So if it's just that you work 12 hours a day, have a long commute, three children to feed and you simply can't be pooped to parade around in a frilly corset for your significant other, you're sane. But if you're *worried* that you're not having any sexual fantasies then you could be insane.

The problem is, many asexuals report feeling distressed, not because they are concerned about not having sex, but because of their struggles to fit in with society. This means that many healthy, otherwise content asexuals are in danger of being handed a mental health label.

In the same way that gay rights activists applied pressure in the 1970s for the diagnostic criteria on homosexuality to be removed from the DSM, asexuality networking group

AVEN has started to push for revised criteria of HSDD. It wants HSDD to be harder to diagnose so that asexuals are not mistakenly pathologised.

Leading the campaign is Andrew Hinderliter, himself an asexual. 'They don't classify asexuality as a disorder *per se* but what we have an issue with is that they lump so many problems to do with desire and libido into one category,' he explained. 'It sends a message to the general public that there is something wrong with not being interested in sex. There are too many factors which contribute to desire – depression, exhaustion, hormones, lack of confidence, having children, age, worry, menopause. Pharmaceutical companies came up with Viagra in 1998 and now they have started to create a drug to fix desire in women, as if it's a singular problem with one single cause. This basically says: "If you're healthy, you'll have a healthy libido", and that isn't necessarily true.'

Sociologist Anthony F. Bogaert produced a prominent piece of research in 2004 which suggested that 1 per cent of the population was asexual. But he himself said that the figure is likely to be higher because by nature asexuals are typically reluctant to answer questions about their sexuality. His research, and subsequent book, *Understanding Asexuality*, prompted the debate as to whether a lack of sexual orientation is down to nature or nurture. The common medical view on homosexuality is that prenatal biological factors control our sexual orientation but with asexuality, experts aren't so sure.

Sociologist Mark Carrigan believes it's nurture. His research into the asexual community left him concerned that a sex-obsessed society is turning many of us off sex.

'There is an intense pressure on young people to sexualise themselves,' Carrigan outlined when I caught up with him.

'As we move from childhood into adulthood there's great emphasis on sexual exploration. Sex is a key step into adulthood. But go back 50 years and this wasn't the case. We've gone from excessive puritanism to a degree of obsession with sex. Children born today have much wider sexual pressures. Many people are not able to manifest the sort of sexuality expected of them and that can be emotionally difficult. This is why we've started to see people identifying as "asexual" – there have always been people who experienced little or no sexual attraction but it's only in recent years [that] it's become problematic and created a need for a group identity so they can say, "There's nothing wrong with me".'

Carrigan conducted interviews and studied hundreds of surveys for his research. He identified a stage at around 15 or 16 years old when sexual pressures from peers kick in for those who feel no sexual attraction. 'I found it striking how marginalised they felt – people described feeling like they were broken, fucked up. They were confused about what was wrong with them. This really raises questions about how we think about sex. Sexual freedom should also mean the freedom to choose not to have sex. It's hard to conceive that homosexuality was once mythical but until we recognised homosexuality, we didn't even have a word for hetero-sexuality. Now that homosexuality has such visibility in society people are confident to own up to it. As asexuality becomes more well known and accepted, I wonder how many people will identify themselves as asexual – I think a lot will.'

It is certainly of concern how much pressure asexuals report to conform to a conventional lifestyle. Singletons are clearly not the only ones who have to hear those cringeworthy words: 'You just haven't met the right person'. Our one-size-fits-all model for relationships has conditioned us to think that sex and love must always go together. For asexuals they clearly don't and throughout history they didn't. It sounds preposterous to suggest that we rethink long-term partnerships as being separate to our sexual needs but evidently many people do. And so do another breed of couple called swingers. Hold on to your keys and cover your fruit bowls because they're increasing in their droves!

CHAPTER 7

Posh Swingers

It was a fittingly dark and stormy night when I arrived at Halswell House, a magnificent Grade I listed seventeenth-century manor house in the Somerset countryside, near the picture postcard town of Goatshurst. My cloak and mask gave me a little protection against the weather albeit not that much for warmth. The wind got right under the cloak and the rain fell in thick cold droplets into the gap at the front, straight through to my scarlet Agent Provocateur two-piece, which was all I had on underneath.

The dress code, you see, had simply stated 'mask & black cape and coloured lingerie (no black)'. So I was following the rules. I arrived via mini cab from the local B&B, which looked a bit pathetic compared to the other guests, who pulled up outside the beacon-lit grand entrance in Porsches and Bentleys, pulling on glittering Venetian masks as they charged purposefully along the gravel path clutching their blustering black cloaks tightly around them.

The location of the party had been kept secret until that

very afternoon to avoid it leaking, such was the level of exclusivity. Two guards dressed in tails and white masks stood by the pillars at the main entrance and guests whispered a password into one of their ears to gain entrance.

I was intrigued but not excited. In my past sugar daddy dating days, when sexual exploration was high on the priority list, I had ticked off a few of these parties already. Saying that, they were always in London and without tonight's fanfare of secret locations and themed costumes so this did have a soupçon of novelty about it.

The party was called 'Eyes Wide Sin', after the 1999 film *Eyes Wide Shut* with Tom Cruise and Nicole Kidman, in which the guests at an imposing mansion engage in an egregious sexual ritual, wearing menacing masks. Strip away the marketing blurb, though, and what you have is a sex party for the middle classes. Posh swinging. It's a bit like getting plastered on fine wines and luxury spirits. You'll still fall over, smell like a tramp in the morning and have a sore head no matter how prestigious the label.

Admittance was by approval only and required a photo application. The organisers, Little Sins, had brought over the parties and much of their impressive guest list from Europe. Based in Amsterdam, they hosted similar parties in Germany, France and Switzerland.

Shane, 33, married for five years, had just taken on the role of organiser of the UK parties. It wasn't his day job, though. In real life he was a buyer for an electronics firm. When I saw him, with his arm draped over three ladies, he was keen to explain how swinging has needlessly got a bad name and how he hopes these elite parties will change that.

'People are much more inhibited in the UK than in Europe, so what you end up with is a hardcore swinging scene where people really go for it. That's why it's perceived as seedy, sweaty basement clubs and desperate men with beer bellies acting like they're on heat. In Europe, people are more liberated so it attracts a more respectable and reserved crowd. It's about meeting a couple you want to go home with.

'There are lots of rules to swinging,' Shane continued. 'All clubs are different but the universal rule is that you always ask if it's OK to join before jumping in. Some couples don't want to swap partners; they just enjoy watching or being watched themselves. Nearly all couples will have some sort of sign, too. For instance, if one presses the other's palm it might mean, "Stop, honey, I'm not comfortable". Or if they stroke their palm, it could mean, "I'm really enjoying this, go for it!" Some women say they don't want their partner to have outright sex with another girl but they put no restrictions on girl-on-girl action.'

There were 300 guests wandering around the maze of rooms in the stately mansion. Door after architraved door opened onto endless oak-panelled lounges and boudoirs, saturated with impressive baroque artwork.

At the stroke of midnight, a loud bell chimed and the guests gathered round a staged re-enactment of the memorable scene in *Eyes Wide Shut* of a hierogamy ritual. Only then, after a priest had chanted something in Latin, could guests remove their cloaks and masks to reveal their skimpies beneath.

My red Agent Provocateur two-piece felt plain in comparison to the lace-rimed basques, diamanté-studded garters, elegant negligées and pink feather boas. Good on the men for going to town, too! While some swaggered around in just black trousers with neatly toned torsos, others wore fishnet body stockings or PVC shorts, and one was in head-to-toe psychedelic rubber, looking a little like he'd gone off route on the Tour de France. A very handsome trim 50-something caught my eye as he padded about in white high-waisted jodhpurs and a crisp white shirt, a silk cravat tightly tucked into his waistband. When I spotted him leaving at 2 a.m., however, it was no longer so crisp and definitely no longer tucked in.

There were restrictions in place, though. Any lustful action was limited to two rooms – the 'couples room' and the 'chill-out room'. The former lay at the top of the grand open oak staircase. It was a huge space with five super-king beds with silky spreads folded back and crisp white sheets waiting to be rumpled. Huge porcelain bowls swimming with shiny packets of condoms were laid on bedside tables at each side of each bed, at the bar, on bookcases and anywhere else with a flat surface. It was hard to walk a few steps without encountering a pick 'n' mix of condoms. The safe sex message in the swinging community is taken seriously. It was emboldened on their (now defunct) website, reiterated in the party email confirmation and backed up again on signs in the ladies, the gents (so I'm told) and on the door of the 'couples room'.

The guests were shy at first. Couples perched upright on the ends of beds, talking to other couples; some of the braver ones ventured for a gentle caress of a hand. But the full-on porn show didn't happen until much later.

I seized my chance to information gather since I suspected that later on, talking might become inappropriate. Nicky, 29, and Harry, 31, were the first to share their story with me. A tall good-looking couple, with strong Yorkshire accents, they had travelled to Somerset from Leeds that morning.

They told me they find parties like these around once every three months. 'It's eroticism without jealousy,' explained Nicky. 'I'd hate it if Harry met someone from work and I found out he'd been for a drink with them, but with this, I don't mind. I can watch him have sex with someone and it turns me on. When we first did it, we had a codeword to say to each other if we felt uncomfortable but we found that we didn't mind seeing the other one with someone else – we loved it!'

'Do you tell people where you're going?' I asked.

'We don't make a point of telling people but we definitely don't deny it,' replied Harry. 'If someone asks me where I'm going, I'll tell them I'm going to a couple's party. I don't say the word "swinging" because it has a pervy image – people think of bald men in steamy clubs which get raided by cops.'

Nicky took over the talking. 'We've been together since we were 15. We're bound to have temptation after all that time – this removes it. We've actually learned more about what we enjoy and what the other one likes. It's made us much more open about sex. We can talk about who we think is sexy, just like you do to your friends. We never could before but I can't imagine not being able to do that with him now.'

My next prey were George and Lillian, a couple in their early 50s. When I approached them, they were clasping hands tightly. I wondered if this was to reassure each other that just because they were considering sleeping with someone else that night, they were still very much devoted to each other. They looked a plain couple. George was short, white-haired, with a square jaw and a ruddy nose. He didn't have the youthful physique for any sort of rubber riggings so he had donned tight-fitting trousers and sported a bare chest and a dog collar. Lillian, in a white negligée, looked nervous and let George do the talking.

'This is our first time at anything like this,' he confessed. 'We've been married for 16 years and never considered opening up. But you know, the kids leave home, you pass milestone birthdays and you start to think, what now? We both felt that we were entering into a new phase of life when the youngest one went to university. We started to talk about what sex would be like with other people. As we talked, it didn't seem such an unreasonable idea so we agreed that if one of us had a fling, the other wouldn't feel threatened. We never did anything about it because I think we were scared that if we were the first, we'd hurt the other or it wouldn't be fair. Then we said, right, if we're going to do it, we have to both do it at the same time. We looked into going to parties where we could meet other couples but they all looked a bit shabby. We considered going to Amsterdam, where it's supposed to have a nicer crowd. As I was researching, I came across this – it's a bit easier to get to than Holland.'

Another younger couple approached me, unprompted. As a writer, I often find people as keen to share their stories as I am to collect them. There is clearly a cathartic reward in articulating thoughts and history. The man introduced himself as Philip. He was good-looking, about 30, with three-day designer stubble.

I was surprised to learn that he was an accountant. His girlfriend Sarah was notably less attractive than him. Despite her large frame she'd decided to opt out of wearing lingerie and had a set painted onto her skin instead. She had dyed burgundy-brown hair. They'd been together since they were 19. 'We've been meaning to come somewhere like this for the last two years but we could never quite bring ourselves to do it,' said Philip. 'We first mooted opening up two years ago – we started to talk about feeling like we might have missed out. We joked about meeting other couples but never did anything about it. Then we talked about going swinging but never did anything about it.

'Around a year ago we met this girl through a mutual friend. She was in the same circle of friends so we kept bumping into her. She started to flirt with both of us. One night we were at a party – I had to leave early and Sarah said, "Would you mind if something happened between us tonight?" Like a typical bloke, I said, "Go for it!" I was quite turned on by the idea. They got it on that night and after that the girl regularly joined us for threesomes. That got us into it so we tried a few parties. This is by far the best crowd we've come across.'

'It was really strange,' said Sarah. 'I didn't think I was attracted to girls but there was something about her. Maybe I thought she was safe because she was a girl and I craved something a bit different after being with Philip for so long. I'm glad it happened. We've been to a few couples parties since then and we love it.'

I noted that Sarah too preferred to euphemise swinging with 'couples parties'. I asked her what the difference was but she couldn't really define it. 'I don't know, "couples party" just sounds nicer,' she said.

With sex, I suppose, it's all about the presentation. Maybe Sarah felt that because these parties come from fashionable Europe they are somehow more refined. Maybe it's vicariously empowering to exchange body fluids with sophisticated members of society. Maybe the decorous surroundings, educated accents, handmade lingerie and chilled champagne in crystal flutes are an intoxicating mix, enabling revellers to lose themselves in erotic fantasy. But if you strip away the velvet coating, you're left with essentially the same thing as goes on in any warehouse sex club.

I'm an immersive journalist and I've always believed experience is the most effective research, but having been to similar themed nights before, I can reliably declare that public sex is not my thing. Needless to say, I remained in my journalistic, observational comfort zone and kept my Agent Provocateur bra fasteners firmly intact. I'll be honest, the sight of a grand, majestic room filled with chandeliers and candles and smooth legs and toned arms tangled together was undeniably erotic; I found it arousing and fascinating. But that's voyeurism and very different to actually mixing sweat and saliva in a hot room with no private en suite to nip into for a quick rinse afterwards.

It may well appeal to some people's fantasies but I'm distracted by the reality, I'm afraid: a bed of alcohol-saturated breath, a whiff of a woman's perfume followed by an aftersmell of the aftershave of the man she was entangled with before you. You'd see beads of sweat and not know if it's theirs, yours or someone you don't know. Definitely not my thing! But as an exercise for couples determined to keep sexual adventure alive, bravo for their chutzpah. At least someone is attempting to tackle the conflict between our thirst for sexual variety and our urge to find a long-term committed partnership.

For Carol and her husband Edward coming to sex parties was a way of detracting from the fact that their own relationship had become platonic. Carol, 45, was a stunning blonde, albeit she might have overdone the Botox. Her thick hair trailed all down her back. 'I'm not really into men,' she purred, looking at me a little too beguilingly for comfort. 'Edward and I have been married for 25 years and I absolutely adore him –' she pointed to a muscular, well-groomed man in a string vest and red leather pants, who was making two girls giggle. 'But he's like my best mate; we're like live-in friends. Sexually I like girls and I just can't pretend to please him any more. He loves that I like girls and he likes watching me with them, but of course he has his own sexual needs and here we can accommodate both.'

'Didn't you know that you preferred girls when you married him?' I asked.

'I knew, but I suppose I never questioned it. I was in love with him and I thought that everyone must dabble with both sexes. No one talked about things like they do today. We were a wild couple and had loads of threesomes – in fact they formed the basis of our sex life. We'd always invite a girl back with us after a party – I thought that was part of the fun of being a wild new couple. I thought our parties and threesomes would last forever. It was only when we got domesticated and I had a daughter and stopped going to parties that I realised I didn't get excited by sex with a man. But we're still in love so why would we change things?'

She was delightfully honest. Like many couples, instead of treating the dwindling limerence in their relationship like the elephant in the room and begrudgingly accepting a sexless marriage, they had evolved with it instead. They had found something that suited their different places in life. Knowing what I learned about romantic orientation in the last chapter, it sounds as if Carol could quite possibly be heteroromantic but homosexual. She was obviously romantically in love with her husband yet she claimed always to have been sexually attracted to women.

Couples made up the majority of the clientele at Eyes Wide Sin but there were a few women who had arrived alone or with friends. One such woman was Lisa, a cute, chatty little thing, brunette and petite, one-quarter Chinese. It was her first time at a party like this: 'I was nervous about tonight but I love it,' she confessed. 'I've watched porn since I was 14 and always felt turned on by it. This is like porn in 3D, like living inside my fantasy. I'm not even attracted to girls, but when someone's girlfriend asked me to join them, I did. It felt amazing to be wanted by two people on both sides of me – I felt adored.'

Men were not permitted to arrive with friends. Single men couldn't be admitted without an accompanying female. Sexist? Maybe, but it's a common rule in all swinger circles, fetish clubs or anything else in the saucy entertainment genre. It's presumably to stop the events attracting swathes of horny men and thus turning off women. A sexually thirsty female is obviously seen as far less threatening than an eager male.

It's a biased rule but if we're honest, we can all see the sense in it. The sociologist Catherine Hakim has put forward a theory in her book *Honey Money*, which she dubs 'the male sex deficit'. She notes that sex surveys around the globe all show men wanting sex more than women, at all ages, and men willing to pay more or risk more to get it. This imbalance between male sexual interest and female sexual availability drives up the value of women's sexuality due to its 'greater scarcity'. In effect, the woman becomes the chooser because her libido needs massaging, but a man's needs reining in. The supply and demand economics explains why single men could not be admitted to the party but single women, who are in more demand, could be. (Of course it also explains why so many men are willing to pay for sex.)

The male sex deficit perhaps also explains why at the Eyes Wide Sin party it was always the women who did the inviting. I was beckoned to join in several *ménages à trois, à quatre* and even *à cinq*! Countless times I was ushered over to one of the super-kings in the couples' room. Each time it was the woman who made the approach – the men waited for the go-ahead from the women. I couldn't help thinking that if the less sexually charged gender is tasked with the decision-making of the sexual agenda, then this free-for-all environment must be potentially quite explosive.

The reason couples treat it so delicately is of course because of the potential for jealousy. Some guests claimed swinging helps jealousy because it allows them to feed their lust in a controlled environment. They made it clear that swinging is not about love but primal urges. Therefore, how could swinging compete with your love for your partner? As the organiser, Shane, put it: 'The ideal partners to play with are couples who are madly in love with each other because they just want fun and there's not going to be any threats.' Still, I suspect jealousy continually lurks around those king-sized beds. The fact that Shane also told me that couples use signs as to whether their partner should continue or stop is another indication of just how hazardous this activity could be.

As the evening came to an end and I stepped outside into the sobering wind and rain, the flaming beacons now nothing but a dull glow, all I could think was, what do these couples do when they go back to their bed & breakfast lodgings? Do they have sex? Perhaps not, as it would remind them that their private sex lives are as humdrum as ever. Or maybe the opposite is the case. Perhaps they do have sex, exclusively, to reassert their intimacy, to expunge the debauchery, to remind each other that what happened in the hours prior was merely physical fun. Or maybe, and probably most likely, they collapse, too champagne-drunk and exhausted to care.

* * *

Swinging isn't such a modern model of relationship. Officially it's been acknowledged for three quarters of a century, but orgies are older than civilisation itself. Rumour has it that swinging started in the Air Force community during the Second World War. Fatality rates for fighter pilots were the highest of any branch of military service and so the surviving pilots took it upon themselves to satisfy the needs of bereft wives.[16]

The idea soon caught on and during the Korean War of the 1950s other military communities adopted the practice. It wasn't long before it spread to non-military society and fashionable parties emerged, where a husband would throw keys into a fruit bowl and select a set at random to decide whose wife he would take home. Or so legend has it. Never was there another era when such louche activities would be so out of place than the 50s, so it wasn't surprising that the media seized upon the underworld trend of having sex with someone else's spouse, referring to it sensationally as 'wife swapping'.

Since then swinging and wife swapping have been

---

16 *The Lifestyle: A Look at the Erotic Rites of Swingers*, Terry Gould. Vintage Books Canada, 1999

associated with squalid clubs in illegal venues in grim city suburbs... until now. For whatever reason, sex parties have started to attract the middle classes. Over the last decade swinging has been creeping onto the landscape of the cultural elite, and the likes of Fever and Killing Kittens have become the poster clubs for a new genre of highbrow sex parties for respectable and fashionable professionals.

Both clubs boast an attractive guest list with an admittance-by-approval policy. Several A-list celebrities have been linked to them and former MP Dougie Smith was alleged to have helped run the Fever club.

In 2009 *The Sunday Times* afforded three pages of glossy coverage to the club Killing Kittens, which was started by the socialite Emma Sayle, a former school friend of the Duchess of Cambridge. It depicted a glamorous, fun-loving crowd, swinging in style. Such a story for a broadsheet newspaper would have been unthinkable 15 years ago.

The idea that we can introduce third parties into our sex lives is quite the rage actually. Actress Cameron Diaz has said she doesn't believe in monogamy. 'Relationships can last two, five or 20 years. I don't believe in sharing your bed with the same person your whole life, though. That might be a reality for some, but it surely isn't for me,' she told the German magazine *Bunte* in 2010. Carla Bruni-Sarkozy also once said she found monogamy boring, before she married the then-President of France. And there have been several big-splash books slating the conservative marital ideal. Even the revered philosopher Alain de Botton says in *How to Think More about Sex* that we shouldn't be so outraged over extramarital nookie; instead of looking at how awful it is when people stray, we should look at how amazing it is that they got so far without straying.

For some open couples, it isn't just sexual appetite that they seek to satisfy. The challenges of long-term commitment can be more complex than things going stale in the bedroom; it can be as much about wanting to love more than one person as lusting after others. These couples want a full, open multi-loving relationship. The poster children for such relationships were Simone de Beauvoir and Jean-Paul Sartre, who met in 1929. Intense lovers and co-writers for 51 years, they never married and remained free to engage openly in other relationships – a radical break from convention at the time. It sounds idyllic, just the sort of passionate, free-from-drudgery affair that I would like to pursue. But are these set-ups so idyllic?

* * *

Now 68, Tuppy Owens has had multiple, loving, open relationships throughout her whole life. As a sexual rights campaigner and organiser of the now world-famous Erotic Awards, she has become a colleague and regular point of contact on any topic to do with laws or campaigns in the sex industry.

Tuppy is passionate about everyone having access to a sex life and has spent much of her life campaigning and raising money for her charity, Outsiders, which helps disabled people socialise, date and have a love life. She runs a sex helpline for disabled people and plays a part in helping them to find sex workers to help meet their needs. She has even formally requested funding from the government for this innovative initiative (to date, they haven't gone for the idea).

When she's not in London trying to persuade health quangos to educate GPs more about sexual health issues,

Tuppy lives in a secluded part of the Scottish Highlands with her younger partner Antony, 50, whom she met 16 years ago.

'I feel strongly about being able to have sex with anyone you like without rules stopping you – life is too short not to,' she opined when I ventured to ask about her open relationships history.

'The rules are that you can't have sex before you know someone well. You can't have sex if you're with someone else. You can't have sex unless you're in love. It's ridiculous. Why?' she asked.

'I suppose people feel threatened by the idea of their partner having sex with someone else because of the emotional side to it,' I suggested. 'They'd be worried their partner may develop feelings for the other person and that's threatening to their love.'

'I think there is more of a danger of people falling in love if they are usually monogamous but have a one-off encounter on the side,' she countered. It would be such a shock to the system they'd probably mistake sex for love because they'd find it overwhelming. That's why you hear about so many idiot middle-aged men who fall in love with their pretty secretaries – they've had one fumble and think they're in love. If we had more sex generally we wouldn't associate sex with love all the time.

'Having multiple partners can be a great thing, and has been a great thing for Antony and I. Most people would appreciate similar experiences if only they could let themselves go and not worry that they're doing something wrong.

'The thought of possessing someone is obscene to me,' she continued. 'Open relationships are generous, sex should be generous – partners are there for you and you want to give them as much pleasure as possible. That means the permission to enjoy other partners. It's an awful thing to do to someone to say they can't have sex with anyone else. If a man hasn't had a partner who allows him to explore sexually with others, it's a great shame. An open lifestyle increases your understanding of the world.

'Very rarely do you get to know someone as you get to know your lovers; you are not having small talk, you are exchanging deep revelations. So many times I've lain in bed and heard a man say, "I've never told anyone this but..." Men in particular feel more comfortable telling a lover something than friends, especially if they are never going to see them again. Maybe that's changed, though. I'm a bit out of touch with very young people.'

Tuppy has never married and never had children. She says matter-of-factly, 'It never happened. I look back now and think, although I'd like to experience childbirth, I'm glad I didn't – what a load of hassle!' I asked her how she first broke the rules with her relationships. Had she always known she had the propensity to love more than one person, like asexuals said they knew their orientation their whole life? Or was it something that she figured over time was a more fitting model to contentment than monogamy?

'One night, when I was in my 20s, I was in this club in London and I ended up pulling a guy I fancied. I started to chat to him and then to flirt a little and I thought, "Gosh this is so easy!" He asked for my phone number and I said, "You don't need my phone number, I'm coming to your hotel tonight!" He couldn't believe his luck. In between sex we talked. He told me he had a disabled daughter and that was the only reason he was still with his wife but he was miserable and depressed.

'A month later I got a letter. He said, "You've changed my life." He said that after our night together, he realised what he was missing. He now goes out with women all the time and has sex. He didn't feel guilty about it any more, he could disassociate it from his duties back home. He was happier and nicer to his wife. I thought, "How wonderful!" I got the man I wanted, we had a good time and it improved his life. With experiences like that, why would I want to stop having sex with people?'

'Does Antony share your view?' I queried.

'Of course. You have to believe in open relationships politically as well as emotionally. If you think politically that everyone can have multiple sexual partners, but then you can't hack it emotionally, it's going to go wrong. But the other way around is more common. Lots of people say they believe in monogamy politically, but physically they can't do it, so they play away. You have to match your beliefs with what you can actually handle. People get all righteous about fidelity, but they can't match their behaviour with their political beliefs.

'I've always had someone special, even though I may have had many lovers at the same time. The person I define as my partner is the one who is my rock. They are the person I need. If I didn't have someone, I'd get panic attacks – I guess I'm a serial non-monogamist!'

When I asked Tuppy if she and her partner still take advantage of the mutually agreed amnesty on fidelity, she smiled: 'When I am away from home, visiting old friends, yes. I think it would be nice to enjoy my time away sexually too. It's part of enjoying yourself. I do find, though, with other men that I don't get the same quality of sex – sometimes in a good way, sometimes in a bad way. It's just different than it is with Antony.'

'Don't either of you get jealous?' I asked.

'I've never looked at a relationship like that. I've enjoyed each experience of different boyfriends at different stages of life. I've never regretted moving on from a man. I just think, "I've met someone else now who fits me better." They have probably thought the same thing about me. It's not a huge issue – people evolve and things change.'

It sounds like one big warm fuzzy love party. But Tuppy's laissez-faire attitude to romantic connections is not without problems. Even she admits that while she was granted freedom by lovers to become an unbounded pioneer, as a woman providing such easy access to sex she was at times left feeling used.

'I've spent a lot of my life upset that I didn't get a phone call the next day. Not because I wanted any more from them than that one night, but because the next day I could still feel them in my body. When I have sex with someone, I have a little bit of love for them. Recently I went to see an old friend in New York. I hadn't seen him for years when he contacted me to tell me he had fallen ill. My first thought was I must go out and see him. Of course he's important to me – I used to shag him!

'I can never understand why people send thank you cards for dinner but not for something so much bigger! I have been terribly upset many times because of the rudeness about sex. You've given someone immense pleasure and they can't even ring up!

'But then,' she added, 'when I have been in a position where I could ring them, I never did either. I couldn't bring myself to. I think it's a case of, "If I ring, they may want to see me again, or they may think I want more and once is enough, so best not." But still, I've always thought sex encounters would lead to more than just a memory – I suppose a friendship or a contact – someone who you think, "I could be useful to that person in the future."'

I am not too dissimilar to Tuppy. Over the past six years I myself have had concurrent lovers. As I so love to mention, I call them 'low-maintenance lovers'. So-named because neither of us have any expectations for exclusivity nor place demands on each other's time, yet we enjoy far more affection, care and consistency than a one-night encounter. We both enjoyed the benefits of intimacy without the monotony and shackles of commitment. The *nouveau* term for these things – a 'fuck buddy' – would be far too derogatory for any of my lovers.

No, I did not want anything more from the sommelier whom I adopted as a summer lover one year, but I still felt connected to him in some way; enough to feel dreadful when I wanted to end it. And the same with a recent American lover I had the pleasure of seeing whenever he hopped on a plane from New York for business appointments in London. No, I'd never choose him as my one-and-only. He wasn't expressive enough for me and he signed his emails with 'cheers' and opened them with 'hi there'. So unattractive! But I still savoured his company and took a genuine interest in his life. We shared an affinity and an exclusive friendship even though I knew it was never going to end with me getting a Green Card.

But like Tuppy, I can attest that casual loverships have their caveats. Non-committal often translates as 'non-caring' and that's a great shame. I learned this when I moved house two years ago. For logistical reasons too complicated to summarise – just go with me – I found myself one night during the move saying to myself: 'If I have two lovers in my life, then why the fuck am I carrying an ironing board, an office chair, three boxes of crockery and two large flat-pack items from IKEA, to whence I have driven a hire car on the very same day as I've cleaned my old flat from top to bottom, an overspilling bag from Homebase, to whence I have also been today, a stone Buddha garden statue which weighs twice my body weight, two bay trees, a projector, a digibox and a stereo down a busy main road at midnight on a frosty January night, from an illegally parked hire car to my stupid new flat, which is still a building site and hence has no place to park?'

How useful it would have been to have had one of those 'low-maintenance lovers' with me at two in the morning, after I'd unloaded everything from said hire car and attempted to return it to the backstreet hire company in my new neighbourhood that I knew nothing about and where I had to wake up the man behind the counter with the car horn because my phone had died (along with Google maps) and then he'd refused to give my cash deposit back because he 'found' scratches on the car. Perhaps if I'd had one of my lovers with me then I wouldn't have burst into tears, lost my temper, threatened to call the police and staged a sit-in to get my money back (all true).

And that's the problem. Casual lovers are appealingly non-demanding but they are fair-weather friends. Few people share the view that intimacy is gradable. For most people love always comes with a capital 'L', or it's just sex. My American lover used to tell me affectionately that he 'loved me with a little l'. Neither of us hid the fact that we viewed our relationship myopically, nor did we let that stop us sharing thoughts, being affectionate, loving each other.

But he was a rare gem. And it's a pity he wasn't in the UK when I needed to transport a concrete Buddha garden ornament across London! Most other dates have either wanted to adopt me as their property or they just like the physical parts. I'm very upfront with any love interests about how I value free time apart and they always say, 'Me too', 'That suits me', 'I'm not demanding'. Or even 'I'll never stop you seeing your friends/going jungle trekking in Thailand/ working on a Sunday'. But then they sulk when you can't take two weeks off and spend two months' worth of salary to go to a Yurt in Iceland for some friend's 40th, who you've never met. Or you go on holiday with them and they feel neglected because you take two hours out to lie in the spa or you want to read for some of the flight. Just speaking from experience...

I find modern values on sexual relations infuriatingly contradictory. We seem to have a marriage-or-fuck approach. On the one hand there is a highly moralising force at play encouraging coupledom: our social welfare system and tax laws reward marriage, insurance companies think people in relationships are less likely to smash up their cars, holiday companies forbid under-occupancy of a room, dinner party hosts only invite couples, middle-aged married women turn their noses up at the gregarious lives of single 'loose' women, and employers favour 'safe' married employees.

People make their approval of long-term relationships very clear. Couples don't get any credit unless they've got the stamp of longevity. 'How long have you two been together?' The longer, the more respectable. Playful new couples aren't 'real' couples. They are merely having a roll in the hay (of which all the marrieds are probably jealous). Yet on the other hand there is a culture that revels in irreverent no-strings encounters. The 'zipless fuck', as writer Erica Jong called it in her cult novel *Fear of Flying*. You don't have to look far to find men and women sniggering about their sexual conquests and boasting of their insouciance for emotional attachment: the cougar who cackles to her single friends how she had a much younger, virile man in her bed for a night, the gutsy student who boasts about 'getting a shag' but not getting his or her number.

Expressing affection or admitting that you're falling for your friend-with-benefits is uncool. The phrase 'love 'em and leave 'em' has become a proverbial high-five among single women comparing pulling notes. Pillow talk is for losers and phone numbers are to be tossed into the bin.

Even teenagers are under pressure to shape their early sexual experiences via a no-strings dynamic. In 2011, research cited in *Psychology Today* found that more teenagers are choosing the 'hook-up culture' over relationships. Children as young as 12 admitted having had casual sex and many of them were apparently going online to look for it. The attitude is widespread among all ages. In another study in 1990, 53 per cent of men and 79 per cent of women considered one-night stands to be wrong. Ten years later those figures had dropped to a third of men and half of women.[17]

To earn one's stripes as a modern independent successful single woman, it seems you have to learn how to have lots of sex and stay disconnected from it. The protagonists in *Sex*

---

17 *Living Dolls: The Return of Sexism*, Natasha Walter. Virago, 2011

and the City conveyed this to their millions of fans. Other female icons of sexual freedom are equally hard-faced. Girl with a One Track Mind and other bloggers write about their glacial sexual experiments; women are told that it's funny not to know his name... unless he's potential husband material, in which case he will be your Prince, your saviour, your soul mate, and you'll move through life together, understand each other deeply, spend every single night of your lives together and live happily ever after. For love rebels like me, who don't view a long-term committed relationship as the elixir of life, we must surely be celibate or a wanton wild child.

In November 2012 the former French Justice Minister Rachida Dati made headlines because it emerged she had eight lovers at the time she fell pregnant with her child. Headlines ensued about her 'dissolute life'. Really? She was dating ministers, TV hosts and a brother of former French President Nicolas Sarkozy. She was having a ball!

Six nights a week with a live-in boyfriend and Sky Plus would probably turn me into a lobotomised tortoise but I bet you my peers and family would give it more of a nod of approval than my current single lifestyle, which is dotted with lovers. I would find zipless fucks equally unsatisfactory, but I would not have to look far to get the thumbs up from a go-getting, girl-power inspired 'liberated' single crowd.

In the 70s, the era that epitomised sexual liberation, icons of the Free Love movement revolved their affairs around passion and emotions, rather than sexual acrobatics. The writer Anaïs Nin celebrated her promiscuity but she always talked about love, as did the novelist Michele Roberts in her memoir *Paper Houses*.

SCREW THE FAIRYTALE

I can't help thinking that this new template for self-gratifying, boisterous, disposable sex has emerged as a backlash to the stringent demands of modern coupledom. True love is daunting. Couples worth their salt go to IKEA together and do up rooms and spend Boxing Day speeding up three different motorways so they can get all the relatives in. Together. We expect nothing less. It goes so much against the trend for autonomy in every other area of the modern world that people want to break away. They want to keep sexual partners at arm's length, lest they overstay their welcome. As Tuppy said: 'You think "I should call", but maybe they think I'll want more so I better not.'

There are many other outspoken commentators who've made this point. In *Living Dolls* the feminist Natasha Walters suggests that the sexual liberation of the 1960s and 70s gave us other things to shy away from. She writes that some women 'feel there is a new cage holding them back from the liberation they sought, a cage in which the repression of emotions takes the place of repression of physical needs.' The French philosopher Pascal Bruckner said in *Paradox of Love*: 'Our parents lied about their morality. Now we lie about our immorality.'

Tuppy found a relationship genre to suit her because she grew up in an era when lovers were celebrated rather than banged against a bedpost and then deleted from a phone. I have struggled to find someone who doesn't want to either see me five times a week or just treat it all as a big jolly. Despite my nonchalant attitude to serious relationships, I quite like the idea of a monogamous lover: exclusive intimacy appeals. But it seems you can only ask for this if you're prepared to give up half your friends, weekend hobbies and your own family Christmases.

When asked to list priorities in their life: relationship, career, home, health, money, etc., no one dares place career above their partner. To them it would be insulting, indulgent, even inappropriate. Well, I do! Very often, I'm afraid I have to admit. When I've been in a relationship, obviously I can recall great shared experiences and laughter but much of the time I can also recall thinking that I'm only spending time at their place because it's part of the weekly relationship maintenance, rather than because I really want to be there.

What I'd really like is a once-a-week relationship. Plus holidays. Not because I want to go off and have sex with other people on the remaining six days (I'd have to get a wax every two weeks and really, who can be bothered?) but simply because I'd like to watch *Newsnight* in peace without someone demanding to know what he's done with his only clean shirt for the morning.

Come to think if it, even during the 'plus holiday' parts, I think it would be very sensible to have an agreement that we do our own things in the day and meet at sundowner hour. I don't know about you but for me there's so much to do even when there's nothing to do. There's the hotel gym, reading the papers, the books you say you'll always read on holiday, the local boutiques to step into. How can I expect a boyfriend to tag along with me while I do all that?!

When you next see a couple on holiday sitting in a café or restaurant, observe them closely: they don't talk. That's because they have nothing to say. They've been together every minute, seen the same things, ordered from the same menu. At least if you're on your own and you have nothing to say, you can always read a book.

All this raises the golden question: is it possible to love

someone fully and loyally without living in each other's pockets, or would you just drift apart? Well, that's where I bring in my favourite type of couple: the committed couples who live apart.

CHAPTER 8

Living Apart Together

The last thing I expected to do while writing a book endorsing singledom and free-wheeling loverships was to fall in love myself. But this was actually a very good thing, not least because it allowed me to see what all the fuss over committed relationships is about. And it enabled me to put my arm's-length-relationship theory to the test. Or more specifically, could I enjoy all the rewards of erstwhile love but still keep a sense of self?

I do recommend falling in love (unless you're already in love because that would be complicated and I would not want to be responsible for the wreckage). Somehow I felt calmer. It was probably all that oxytocin running through my system, which we apparently get from human touch and affection and.... ssshhh... sex! I found myself smiling at strangers and making jokes with shop assistants even when I'd had to queue for ages.

We'd known each other professionally for two years but I was too busy writing about how I liked being single to notice him. He was a freelance PR and as such had regularly contacted me suggesting stories about his clients. I'll let you into a secret. When I first knew him, I found him a real pest. '*What does he want now*?!' I was tiring of short-term lovers but I still had no interest in anything more permanent or demanding. It was as good as a man detox. But he pursued me graciously. Each email was laced with a witty comment or a thoughtful observation and he never forgot anything I'd previously told him. Slowly I found my irritation softening until one day I found to my surprise, that I found myself looking forward to his wittering emails, wondering what funny observations he'd have to say this time.

It all progressed very quickly. Even before the first week was up, he'd suggested trips away or visits to friends in overseas places. By week two we'd met at least two of each other's friends. Then by week three I'd done half of all the coupley things that I usually roll my eyes about. Yet as much I was enjoying this novel feeling of falling in love and being loved, I was troubled by what I would lose. Six years of utilising the opportunism of singledom had made for a full schedule and there wasn't much I wanted to cross off. So it was only fair that I shared these concerns. If he were looking for a five-times-a-week girlfriend, I had to make it clear that I was never going to be one. Better to knock down unrealistic expectations before they get unmanageable. So I told him how much I value time alone, the luxury of spontaneity and how strongly I feel about maintaining space for friendships and other of life's interests.

He too had been single for several years so he related. He even joked that being my first proper boyfriend in all this time meant he had a responsibility to restore my faith in relationships; he was determined to show me that relationships could be more rewarding than crowding. But I had to be double-triple sure. So I brought up the issue of children: 'I am not going to change my mind about wanting them. Are you sure you are OK with that?' I phrased it in different ways, thinking I was cleverly disguising the question just so I could be sure. Had he ever felt sad he hadn't had kids? Had he ever felt the need to leave his DNA footprint on the earth? Really subtle things like that! I wanted to make absolutely sure that I would never find myself being unwittingly persuaded into a life of school runs further down the line. And I never wanted to deal with the guilt of robbing a broody man of his chance to have children.

I was all assured. In fact, he observed that before he had met me he had never questioned taking the marital route in life. He had just assumed that's what would happen. Now he realised he had options and that was comforting. And then, just I was starting to relax into a nice, low-impact twice-a-week routine, I got my first niggle.

We were at his home – a lovely house in a leafy part of London suburbia. He was talking me through some of the work he had done to his house and what else he wanted to do. There had been the snazzy kitchen extension, the office in the garden. Then, moving on to the plans for his guest room – as if he had forgotten who he was talking to – he said, 'I've always thought that a girlfriend would move in and make this into a dressing room and walk-in wardrobe.'

A little jolt of worry went through me then, which later settled into a niggle that never quite went away. I may well have let myself fall rip-roaringly in love but the single aspect that I most value about my current life is the liberty that comes from living alone. I love everything about it, from the sound of my handbag dropping to the floor in an empty hallway to being able to stick the same spoon into things that I've eaten from. Nothing else about adapting to coupledom had troubled me yet. I'd even unflinchingly foregone a few morning runs in the name of a lie-in with my lover. I didn't mind packing my overnight bag and earplugs once a week to go and stay with him and I'd even cleared him some wardrobe space for the times he stayed with me. This whole relationship thing hadn't been anywhere near as intrusive as I had feared... until he said that.

A walk-in-wardrobe may be some women's empyrean but it wouldn't be my empyrean in *my* house. Having a guaranteed, tranquil, secure, clean, personalised living space gives me more contentment than anything else. But now I felt this would come under threat if things kept hurtling ahead at the speed they were. I was scared that I might slowly, step-by-step, forget how happy it makes me to live alone and I'd get sucked into a gulf of domestic routine and DVD box sets. It's always harder to hold onto your own personal values if they're not conventional ones. 'One day,' I thought, 'there's going to be a conversation about moving in and I'm going to have to somehow articulate why maintaining my own space is so very integral to my sense of wellbeing, without sounding as hippified as that just did.'

If I were to list all the little things that I like about living alone, they would sound futile, but when I add them up it's everything about my daily life. If, for instance, I were to attempt to say that I love my morning routine, I would essentially be saying that I'd prefer to wake up to John Humphries in the morning than him.

So strong was my niggle that I was having imaginary arguments. I'd say to friends, 'But I don't *want* a walk-in wardrobe in a four-bedroom house with a man I love!' No one would understand why I was putting up such a fuss. They'd tut and tell me not to be silly and before I knew it, I'd crumble. I'd be living in someone else's home, where the heating is never on, blokey guests stay until three in the morning, neighbours bring their moulting dogs round and someone will have drank the last of the Innocent smoothies just when I'm the most hungover I've ever been in my whole life. So persistent was this niggle that the next morning, when I had a shower in his bathroom, I looked up and thought: 'It's a *rain* shower. I could *never* live with anyone who doesn't have a detachable shower head.'

So what is the answer? Throw away a loving, wonderful man so that I can sometimes eat porridge for tea? Thankfully not! It's now not so uncommon for perfectly loving committed couples to choose to live apart on a long-term basis. They are part of a fast-growing demographic known as LAT – Living Apart Together.

* * *

The term LAT is not a trendy media phrase. It was first used by the Office for National Statistics in its winter report of 2006. The report estimated that two million people are LATing, which works out at three in every 20 people aged between 16 and 59, about the same as those cohabiting.

Some of that figure will no doubt be new couples who consider it too soon to live together or those who want to live together but circumstances don't allow them to do so. Even so, the figures certainly show that commitment does not automatically go hand in hand with cohabitation. The polls say as much. A British Social Attitudes survey of 2006 found that 54 per cent of people agreed that 'a couple do not need to live together to have a strong relationship' and only 25 per cent disagreed. In another survey on sexual attitudes by the University of Oxford in 2000, one fifth of people aged 16–44 described 'living together apart' as their 'ideal relationship'.

Such is the interest in this new vogue that in April 2013 the Economic and Social Research Council put together a substantial piece of research into whether LAT living might be a way of sustaining intimate relationships in the twenty-first century. It interviewed more than 600 LAT couples, of whom 30 per cent were LATing by choice. Its key finding was that LATs are young: 61 per cent are under 35 and another 28 per cent between 36 and 55. More evidence, I think, of an emerging generation that favours independence over the fairytale.

Also significant was the fact none of the LATers interviewed said they viewed themselves as consciously shaping an alternative lifestyle. Sexual exclusivity was still a must for nearly 90 per cent of them and there was an overall high level of satisfaction with their relationships. So much for the fairytale doctrine that love always leads to a shared doormat.

Celebrities have been way ahead of the LAT trend. In the sought-after location of Primrose Hill in north London, Tim Burton and Helena Bonham Carter have houses next door to each other. A similar arrangement was adopted by Woody Allen and Mia Farrow, who famously lived on either side of Hyde Park. Simone de Beauvoir and Jean-Paul Sartre at one time had separate apartments in the same street. Chef Rick Stein and his partner Sarah Burns take this a few steps further and are on opposite sides of the world, he in Cornwall, she in Sydney. Singer Natalie

Imbruglia and her Australian rock star husband Daniel Johns have a similar trans-hemisphere commute: she's in London, he's Down Under. 'He's got so many more songs written in the weeks he's been away from me,' she has been quoted as saying.

Even more apart than that are Toyah Willcox and her husband of 12 years, guitarist Robert Fripp. They claim they get one month a year together. 'We're never bored with each other, just always thrilled at the thought of meeting up again and leaping into each other's arms,' she told the *Independent* in 2006.

It says something that the key trendsetters for separate living spaces are celebrities. One assumes they have greater financial means than the rest of us to live apart. They are also more likely to have busier and more varied lives and probably a greater need for flexibility and solitary down time. At least that's how it works for me. The busier I am, the more I want time to myself when I shut my front door. For most of us, there are two things that would hold us back from LATing: money and the stigma of breaking away from custom. Celebrities are less likely to have cause for concern in either of those departments, which makes me think that those who can live apart, do.

That's certainly the case for Gillian, 61, and her husband Ryan, 62, both teachers. They lived next door to each other for several years and Gillian claims it saved their marriage. They would have liked to keep things that way but when Ryan retired two years ago, they could no longer afford it.

They began to live apart eight years ago after Ryan was made redundant. According to Gillian, he became withdrawn and difficult. Gillian said that he had always been 'a bit of a bully' and she had always put up with it but after his redundancy things worsened.

'Everything had to be his way. He could behave quite badly if he didn't get what he wanted. He drank and smoked, and I would go a long way to make sure he had cigars to smoke. If he had his way he'd be calm and I'd feel calm.

'A few months after his redundancy, he dropped out of a weekend away with another couple and I remember feeling so relieved that he wasn't coming. That was the signal to me that I didn't want this anymore. Up until then I had been living my parents' marriage. They had a post-war, stiff-upper-lip, male-dominated marriage and so I just took it, thinking that's normal, but after that realisation about the holiday, I said, "No more".'

Ryan was sent on his way and spent weeks at friends. Gillian was adamant he wasn't coming back. He begged, she refused. Then the terraced house next door became available and it seemed a good halfway point between taking care of each other and total estrangement. 'When you've been married to someone for 25 years you still want to help them,' Gillian explained. She firmly believed that once he learned to overcome the emotional turmoil of his redundancy, they would part for good but they soon discovered that separate addresses solved everything.

'Living with a wall between us made a huge difference. The bullying transformed overnight. I realised just how controlling and self-centred he had been all these years. I hadn't noticed the dynamic at the time; now I saw my whole life in a new light.

'When he moved out, it felt like being liberated from a straitjacket. In a marriage people regard you as a mirror image of each other, as a half of one thing. That was always an unsatisfactory reflection for me.

'I got married at 21 so I had been "Mrs" for all that time. Now I detached myself from the status of "Mrs". It was liberating, it was wonderful! I felt like I was taking up residence in my own house. I had choices. I could decorate it how I wanted and get rid of his things I didn't like.

'By living apart you keep control. Our relationship had very good things about it but those things were overshadowed by the routine I had created around him. I found myself doing more activities. When you're on your own you don't think twice about popping out. With someone else at home, organising anything is like playing a three-legged race – you have to coordinate everything. My sleep improved too. I now can't bear to be in the same bed as him. When we go to see friends they put us in the same bed, and it isn't comfortable at all!

'He didn't like the fact that he was relinquishing control. He wanted very much to move back in together. He made fumbling efforts, taking me for dinner and buying champagne, which for him is a big thing because he's tight as anything! It didn't cut much ice, I have to say: now that I had my freedom I wasn't going to back down.

'My friends started to come over a lot. They never did before because Ryan didn't like it. I hosted a big party once. Ryan hated it; he emerged from his house and knocked on the door and told us to keep the music down. I rolled my eyes and told him to stop being so grumpy. I never could have had a party when we lived together. We never even had dinner parties – he says he feels intimidated by guests.'

The benefits of living separately paid off for Ryan too because gradually the hostility between him and Gillian melted and they began to spend more time with each other. 'He had a key and each morning brought me a cup of tea. At weekends I'd go over and say, "Do you want to do something today?" Sometimes we had something on, sometimes not. We cherry-picked the events we did together. It was like having a really good friend next door, who you can ask to come with you to things and tell them to go away when you've had enough of them. And he was still there for practical stuff. When my car goes wrong I find it terrifying, so he still dealt with it. We had the best bits of marriage and none of the horrible bits.

'In the beginning I did have my moments where I felt lonely and vulnerable. I remember getting a pang of envy when someone told me that every Friday they get a Chinese takeaway with their husband. I'd think, how lovely to have that security. But I soon adapted.

'I now regret that I didn't do the things I now enjoy in my earlier years of marriage. When you've been married for 30 years you don't recognise the habits you form. I didn't see how I'd tiptoed around him and put my needs last. We see it in other people, don't we? But we never say anything. It's the thing your best friend sees but doesn't tell you.'

Ryan soon found a new job and the pair lived happily next door to each other for eight years. But then he took retirement and with a dramatically reduced income, they were forced to give up the property next door. Ryan had to move back into the main abode with Gillian.

'I was very disappointed,' said Gillian. 'If I were rich, I would instigate a similar arrangement in a flash. Money is still the biggest thing that makes people live together. When I told anyone about our living arrangements, their first comment was usually about the affordability of it. Everyone could see why it made sense. Most probably they wanted the same themselves, but it comes down to affordability.'

Gillian and Ryan have now been living together again for two years but they keep separate bedrooms and Gillian says the balance of power has changed for the better. 'Living apart makes love blossom more. You become known for who you are, not as the shadow of your spouse. It was a luxury. At the end of each month there wasn't much money left but that's the way the cookie crumbles. We stretched our budget but it was worth doing because our marriage is different now.' Then she added with a wry smile: 'It's also amazing how tidy he has become now that he's had a place of his own!'

Gillian and Ryan were able to maintain daily contact because there was only a brick wall and three yards separating them. But what about LAT couples with several miles between them? My new 'boyfriend' (it still feels strange to write that word and I would prefer 'medium-maintenance lover' but it doesn't roll off the tongue well at parties) lives 15 postcodes away from me and I'd be quite happy to keep things on a once-or-twice-a-week basis. But can long-distance LATing couples still maintain their intimacy?

Olivia, 61, and Alan, 58, seem to do so. They don't live apart because of domestic minutiae but because they have vocations and family commitments in different countries and why should an incidental thing like a partnership make you abandon them? The pair met at art college in their late twenties but didn't marry until 10 years later when their first daughter was born. Olivia is originally from Israel and Alan is English. After several years living in London before children, they moved to the Netherlands for Alan's work.

After 18 years, as the first of their two children left for university Alan was made redundant. Unable to find work in the Netherlands, he had luck in the UK and so didn't hesitate to relocate. By then Olivia was already established in her own career as a fashion buyer in the Netherlands. For her, moving countries was out of the question.

'I wasn't going to give up my life and live in a little cottage in the English countryside!' she scoffed loudly, with a great big rounded flick of her hands. 'I'd probably jump off the roof after a week! Village life is not for me – I need to be in the centre of a town. It's lovely and I go there to visit Alan and so do my daughters, but living there was out of the question.' A larger-than-life character, Olivia is beautiful, glamorous and voluptuous. She talked at one hundred miles an hour and adorned her strong opinions with vigorous gesticulation.

'At first it was a culture shock since we'd always lived together but we got used to it very quickly. I was busy with my own work – I travel to China, India and all of Europe – so there wasn't much time to think about it. Now I really enjoy living apart. I have always enjoyed my own company and now even more so. Most of my friends in Holland are single women – some divorced, some never married, some widowed – all sorts.

'I think we have the ideal marriage actually. I highly recommend that at a certain stage in life people do this. You get old, he snores, she farts – everyone wants to have their own space. Definitely separate rooms anyway!'

I asked Olivia if the 300 miles of separation made their marriage more romantic and she almost spat her coffee out, snorting with laughter. 'No, it's same old! Romantic love is a flash in the pan. What you want with marriage is a friend for life. All this business of romance would embarrass me – that's for my daughters.'

But has it at least strengthened their friendship? 'I wouldn't say that,' she answered thoughtfully. 'If you live apart there is a chance you will grow apart. You get used to being on your own; you get your own sets of friends. It is more friendly between us, though – we don't annoy each other and we have lots to say when we see each other but I wouldn't say it has improved us.

'When we lived together we were closer, obviously. But the whole relationship was different. We were younger, we had children; we were an organised family. There was a routine, dinners were on the table every evening; there was more responsibility. In many ways it is easier for me now. I was always the organiser in our relationship and that could be hard. Alan is laissez-faire and he prefers me to make the decisions for the family.'

'Do you miss him?' I asked.

'Sometimes, but not often. I miss the family meals, especially Fridays when we'd all relax together afterwards. We both love art and we used to go to museums and exhibitions together. I do that less now. But then we can keep in touch so easily because of Skype. Maybe when we retire we'll live together again but we still have this question of where? My friends keep asking me this and I just don't know.'

When I asked Alan, separately, how LATing has changed their relationship, his responses were a beautiful reflection of Olivia's views, with just the nuance of differing personalities. A gently spoken man, he was tall and skinny with a beard and a warm openness about him. 'I never would have asked Olivia to come with me – she had her own work and friends, and everything else,' he told me. 'It wasn't such a big thing for us because we've always had a great deal of respect for each other's space. We were lucky we had a big house in Holland with our own offices to work in. Olivia would disappear off upstairs, do whatever – listen to music – and then come down several hours later, and then disappear again. I did the same.

'Even when we were living together and the children were small, we weren't the quintessential married couple who were always together. Maybe it's because we are arty types and independent-minded. When I listen to people at work talk about their spouses I sense an incredible amount of bickering. They seem not be able to leave each other alone; they seem to be conscious of what the other is doing all the time. But we never had that – I never sat around wondering what my wife was doing.'

Alan hadn't always been so single-minded. He grew up in a small town and always believed he would have a conventional marriage – get together, stay together, grow together – until he met Olivia, who had other ideas. 'When we had been dating for a year or so, she just said one day she had a job in New York and off she went for eight months. I was left behind in London, working away,' he laughed. 'I wasn't happy about it but I thought I'd better get used to it if I wanted to stay with this girl. And then I thought, "Actually this is quite exciting." I had the opportunity to go to New York and then to other places because she was often travelling or going back to Israel to visit family. Being from a different culture she was different to anyone I'd ever met. I got to see fascinating countries and meet fascinating people.' He added with a smile: 'Maybe I had to go through the pain barrier of missing her but I've certainly grown into this lifestyle.'

'How has living apart changed the dynamic between you?' I asked, admiring the fondness with which he spoke of Olivia.

'I have a lot more respect for her. When we lived together in Holland we saw each other every day and if I compare it to that, I look at her differently now. That sounds like I didn't respect her before. That certainly isn't true but it's just that we are not in each other's skin all the time and we notice each other more.

'The downside is that I have to think for myself more. Men are just not as good at organising their lives as women are,' he smiled again. 'But in other small ways it's good. I find myself doing things that I wouldn't do normally – like reading more, listening to more music, watching more movies. I find activities. I'd prefer to have her around me, given the choice, but I also like what we have.'

One of the hardest things to deal with for Alan and Olivia was not the being alone but being accepted by friends.

'We get a lot of raised eyebrows,' Olivia told me. 'People can't fathom it. They look at me suspiciously and ask why. Then they whisper, "Are you separating?" I have to say, "No, we just live apart." It's nothing more complicated than that but some people think I'm covering up. Perhaps they even want me to be covering up because they are jealous. I think they're jealous because there are others who say we have the ideal marriage and they wish they had our set-up too.'

Alan was equally exasperated by others' views: 'The people in the village are all very well-to-do. They think it's all a bit odd. I don't have a close-knit family – I see them occasionally and I think they think we've separated. Being English they don't ask it, but I can feel that they think it. My best friend from school is a bit like me – a free spirit – and he has no issue. He says, "That's typical you." But less close friends think it's odd and they are embarrassed about talking about it. But then there are others who make envious noises. One woman recently said, "I bet you really like having no one watching over you." It was almost a mocking comment, but there was a reflection of her own envy there. A few others have said, "It must be really nice that you can do what you want on your day off." They're small meaningless comments but it obviously reflects the things they feel they can't do, because they watch over each other.'

It's exactly the fact that Alan and Olivia *don't* watch over each other that sets them apart from other couples. It seems the only reason they can tolerate the distance between them while other couples can't is their lack of jealousy. Both consider the idea of finding a new lover preposterous.

'I don't think I would have an affair!' Olivia exclaimed incredulously. 'I couldn't be arsed! It's too much hassle. Men are baboons anyway. Who wants it? It's just not worth it!' Nor does she show a hint of insecurity or possessiveness that her husband may get up to no good on the other side of the North Sea. 'I don't feel jealous in the least!' she snorted. 'Not in the least! If he suddenly tells me, "Look, I've got a girlfriend", maybe I'll feel different, but I don't lie awake worrying about it. He's not the type. His life is very frugal – he lives in the country, he rides bikes and plants trees. He's an antisocial type.

'Even my friends say, "Don't you worry he's having an affair?" As if they expect it. Just because I'm not there, someone else doesn't have to be! I wonder why I do not feel as jealous as them? I think it's because I know that I could survive alone if something did happen.' Almost as an afterthought she added, 'But then you never know. There's always a chance that anyone might meet someone when they're on their own because they feel they need someone. It would surprise me but it wouldn't kill me.'

So does Alan feel equally confident in his wife's assurance that 'men are baboons' or does he secretly wonder how she spends her evenings in the Netherlands or Israel?

'I suppose if there is one worry, that would be it,' he answered. He had a lovely way of speaking that assured his listener he was speaking from the heart. 'But then I've always told myself that if it happens, I can't do anything about it. If it happened there would be a reason – either I'm inadequate or she's gone off me. This long period apart may become a reason but it is out of my control. Other couples keep each other in each other's sights because they feel they possess their partner but I think it is wasted energy to worry about it.'

'Do you worry about yourself straying?' I probed.

'Physically, it is a difficult thing to handle,' he admitted. 'Maybe this is why I do so much fitness as a form of physical release. I don't deny that it could happen but I'm not looking for it. I'm a routine person, I can amuse myself easily; I like people and like talking, but I don't seek activity. I can't see how I'd find it if I wasn't looking.'

* * *

Alan's last comments confirm what I suspected – that most couples don't want to live together so that they can gaze into each other's eyes over their cereal every morning, but because it brings their partner more tightly into their possession. It seals off the distractions and the temptations from the big bad outside world. Living together makes each other more accountable and so it becomes harder to leave.

I always read online comments on newspaper articles because I think they provide a representative window into the opinions of the masses. LATs regularly appear on feature pages, such is the cultural appetite for finding new, more harmonious ways of conducting relationships. Interestingly, the comments that are critical of LAT lifestyles are mostly based on the argument that living apart would give one partner carte blanche to sleep around. 'Good idea, but when the cat's away…' wrote one. Those in favour of it were along the lines of: 'Lucky them! If only we could afford to do that'. Also summed up well by one frustrated married friend, who said to me recently, 'I just don't like living with a man!'

Personally I think LATing is the closest I'll ever get to solving my conundrum of wanting love but valuing my independence more. But the biggest problem I face is the reactions of everyone else. I don't think it's the case that most of us find separate living arrangements unappealing, it's more that we find it threatening. When the media reported on the increasing numbers of solo dwellers, commentators jumped on the 'this is evidence of a fragmented society' bandwagon again.

In case you are wondering, there are nearly 3.5 million people over the age of 45 living alone in the UK according to government statistics. This figure has grown by more than 50 per cent since the mid-1990s. In 1950 only 10 per cent of British households consisted of only one person. In 2012, 29 per cent of homes were registered as single-occupancy.

One right-leaning newspaper reported on these statistics when they were released in November 2012, referring to 'the appalling figures' that signified an 'epidemic of loneliness'. It quoted a family researcher calling for the government to take action to halt the change.

Yet the rise in single people or those who live alone is natural progression in a society that is becoming more autonomous. According to the sociologist Eric Klineberg, single people and those who live alone are twice as likely as married people to go to clubs and bars, more likely to eat out in restaurants and more likely to take art or music classes, or go to public events. As Klineberg says in *Going Solo*, people are choosing to live alone because they can. He opens his book by highlighting the magnitude of this change: 'Human societies, at all times and places, have organised themselves around the will to live with others, not alone. Until now. During the last half century our species has undergone a remarkable experiment. For the first time in human history great numbers of people at all ages in all places from all political persuasions are beginning to settle down as singletons.'

Scandinavia has the highest number of single households in the world at 40–45 per cent depending on the individual country, but it has more space, lower property prices and one of the most generously funded childcare systems in the world. It seems to me that people in those nations live alone because it is viable.

In the early months of my new 'proper relationship', everyone asked whether we had plans to move in. When I say everyone, I mean *everyone*. Even my sports masseuse got her hopes up when I told her about the stirring in my love life.

'So it's serious?' she asked excitedly.

'I suppose it is.'

'Do you think you'll move in?'

She sounded shocked when I said, 'No way!' It's as if cohabiting is a marker of success. To validate our love we have to uproot our entire lives, even if they were completely sorted before. Love has to gobble up your life and if it doesn't, it's not 'serious'. The sports masseuse double-checked the next time I saw her: 'Still no plans to move in?'

I had no idea just how much of a milestone cohabitation is considered to be until I found myself in a relationship. It disturbs me to think that love can't be validated unless it ultimately leads to a shared front door. First, why the rush? It had only been four or five months and now everyone was on the edge of their seats for us to leave our own homes and start a new one. (Do they think we still live with our parents and don't have a sofa to snog on?) Second, why move in ever, unless you're about to have kids? Unless watching one's partner clip one's toenails and shave one's legs in the bath is sexy, I'm puzzled as to what people think it will achieve.

When I walked home from the 'proper boyfriend's' house one Sunday night around a year into our relationship, I passed a house just as a man was turning the key in the lock, his arms full of shopping. As he stepped inside, I could hear children's laughter and the sound of the TV; I could sense a buzz of activity. That was his home. As he disappeared inside, I imagined a warm kitchen and him taking the contents out of the bags and the kitchen slowly filling up with the smells and sounds of family life. Good for him! He looked happy. But I did not think longingly, 'I wish I was going home on a Sunday night to a kitchen filled with the smell of cooking and the sound of human voices'. I thought, 'Thank God I'm on my way home to an empty flat, where I shall kick off my shoes, put on some music to suit my mood, read one of the five books I have on the go, and go to bed at whatever time my eyes start to close, free from anyone's mindless chatter and without their sticky little mitts on my kitchen units!' One person's loneliness is another's paradise.

In the same way, some people's paradise is sharing your love nest with 17 people. Seventeen polyamorous lovers, to be precise! Yes, that's my version of hell, but nevertheless it's where I'm taking you next.

CHAPTER 9

My Fifteen and Only

The three times I've been to Scotland I have always had to buy a new coat on arrival. As soon as I stepped out of Waverley station, my overnight bag stuffed with a clean pillowcase, towel and warm pyjamas, an icy wind ripped through me. I was fearful that the commune where I would be spending the night (gulp!) might not have central heating, so I found a Primark and bought a mac to be on the safe side.

After a half-hour wait I was eventually greeted on a cold drizzly street corner by a stranger in a 4x4 called Dan, with long, greasy ginger hair and a goatee. Dan had been sent by his wife Tania to pick me up and bring me to their shared commune in a village in Fife, an hour north of Edinburgh. I had met Tania in my duties as a judge at The Erotic Awards. She was one of the performers and had told me about her nonconventional home life as we talked backstage. When I told her that I was writing a book on alternative relationships, she invited me to stay a night.

When I say nonconventional, what I mean specifically is that she is in a relationship with 17 people. Yes, 17! Dan was currently the only man but that hadn't always been the case. Not that gender mattered because everyone in the relationship was bisexual and loved each other equally and unreservedly. The name for this ability to love more than one person is polyamorous.

I was mildly apprehensive about my one-night sojourn as we drove over the Firth of Forth. What exactly does a commune look like? Where would I sleep? If this crazy-sounding group ever went to bed at all, that is. And if I did get a bed, or an old mattress or something, what if it was some damp, dirt-encrusted used bedding? For the fifth time that day, I commended myself for remembering to pack my own pillowcase (thanks, Mum, for that life lesson).

On arrival I discovered their polyamorous lair was in fact a modest and immaculately clean five-bedroom house. Bricks and mortar was a great relief – I had feared the commune might be a collection of campervans and caravans, perhaps even a tent, and the shower would be an outdoor tap with a hose on the end, as is the enduring image from younger years spent backpacking on a shoestring.

There were even flower boxes by the front door. On the walls of the porch hung photos of what looked like Pagan handfasting ceremonies. A younger and slimmer version of Dan featured in several of them, with different brides in brightly adorned Edwardian gowns and furs. There were photos of female couples too. Some smiled for what looked like a civil wedding ceremony while others posed in the midst of dancing circles around trees.

'Those are our wedding photos,' confirmed Dan. Later I learned that there were several overlapping marriages within the group (some were legally married to one partner and had affirmed Pagan partnerships with others). Dan had been legally married to Tania, whom I had begged, pleaded and buttered up for access to this place, for 20 years but was also betrothed to four more of the women through non-legally binding Pagan handfastings. That left 12 women in the group whom he hadn't married, but that didn't mean he didn't love them as much. 'Sometimes it feels right to marry and sometimes it doesn't,' he had explained during our journey there.

I was escorted into the kitchen and was overwhelmed by the warmth of my reception. The room was filled with heat from an AGA and the comforting smell of slow cooking. A sea of young, fresh, female faces smiled up at me from where they were sitting on wooden chairs around a large pine dining table.

It was only 5 p.m. but it was clear that what was bubbling away on the stove was to be served imminently. This was dinnertime. I pulled up an uncomfortable wooden chair – the type I used to sit on in school assemblies – and joined them. Tania was nowhere to be seen.

'Tania is whacked out on morphine upstairs, bless her,' said a girl with long, mousy-blonde straggly hair called Chrissie, as if she could read my mind. It wasn't what you think – Tania had emailed in advance to tell me that she had hurt her back and the only position she was able to adopt was standing or lying on her front.

Other house members started to trickle in, drawn by the smell of dinner. Three emerged stark naked, looking sleepy. They held out limp hands to introduce themselves as Isobel, Katie and Amanda. For the rest of the evening they didn't bother to put any clothes on. They plonked themselves down on the wooden chairs alongside their clothed housemates as though they weren't even aware that their buttocks were bare. I had a lot to take in but during dinner all I could think was, 'I hope they clean the chairs with antiseptic wipes!'

The group was noticeably tactile. Often, as two of them crossed paths, they'd pause to kiss, sometimes a full-on snog; other times just a touch of the lips. It was done lackadaisically, as if a programmed mark of affection. Two girls, Fran and Suzy, sat in a tight embrace for the entire duration of the evening; it was as if they'd fall over if they let go.

Dinner was curry. There were three different varieties served in three big pots on the kitchen worktop and a selection of naan, rice and Sainsbury's Taste the Difference poppadoms, which I thought was a nice take on their anticapitalist leanings. They all got up from their seats and formed an orderly queue around the worktops.

'I remember you from the Erotic Awards,' giggled a girl with long mousy, straggly hair. She was childlike, yet looked to be in her late 30s and exuded a mischievous energy. She soon became my favourite because of her regular quips and witty comments followed by bursts of giggles. I, of course, did not have the faintest memory of whom she was.

'It's Rachel,' she reminded me, much to my relief. 'Lillie always cooks,' she went on. 'And she clears up. She does all the cleaning and the house chores – she likes to.'

The girl stirring the curry on the AGA turned round and smiled seductively. I think I even caught her looking at my chest! She was wearing jeans with the top button popping open and a white T-shirt that had gone a bit grey. 'When people visit the house, they get really freaked out by the fact that I do all the cooking and cleaning. Because I'm Asian, it makes people really uncomfortable. It goes with the Asian stereotype, doesn't it, that we are the servants who do all the domestic work?' she mused.

I gave a half-nod, not knowing what to say. The fact that she was Asian and cooking did not appear to be incongruous to me at all. 'But I like doing what I do,' she continued, as if she needed to convince me out of a judgement that I hadn't made. 'Everyone has a role in the house. Some of us go to work. Amanda, Kitty, Isobel and Fran go out painting and decorating, and Dan has his film-editing business. Some of us do practical things, like managing the bills or looking after the garden. But me, I like doing the cooking and cleaning.'

'We can't even make a cup of tea!' laughed Dan. 'If someone wants a cup of tea, I get it for them,' agreed Lillie. 'It's my kitchen!' And she laughed.

We started to eat in silence. I felt their eyes on me, waiting for me to ask them questions. They were well aware that they were my research subjects but their expectancy was unsettling. I soon learned that out of the 15 in the relationship, 10 had been together for nearly 20 years, joining Tania and Dan shortly after they got married. Another 10 had joined and left over the years, and the current members had more or less been the same for the last eight years with only one new face, which was Isobel. Two people had left within the last year. There was a man who wanted to go travelling and a girl who left to get married, ironically to a wealthy, well-to-do older man. There had been one birth, 10 years ago, but Dan denied being the father. They were living in Andorra at the time in a similar set-up. Mother and child remained with the group for three years, but then the mother wanted to place her daughter in the UK schooling system. Dan, Tania and the rest of the group claimed they didn't mind a baby living with them, but reading between the lines it seemed they were relieved when the mother and her crate of toys departed: 'None of us in here are into children,' Lillie stated firmly. 'We all feel the same, which makes things easier. It also makes sense that we all take the Pill at the same time and then we're in synch hormonally.'

So how on earth did the original 10 get together in the first place?

'Tania always liked girls,' Dan explained. 'I didn't mind her having flings with girls but she always fell in love with them. She started to include me in them and once I realised that I was allowed to love them, it became remarkably easy to love more than one person and just all be together. I can't imagine only living with one person now.'

Neither their landlord nor their neighbours knew the dynamic, believing the four-bedroom property housed four couples. 'We do have some friends outside of our relationship, but mainly people we've known a long time who accept us. Most people can't understand how we live, so it's easier to keep it to ourselves,' said a girl called Bettina. She too had long, mousy, straggly hair – it was hard to tell them apart.

They were defensive about Dan being the only male, going to great lengths to put paid to any assumptions that the household was a male-controlled harem. 'When people come into the commune, they presume that I must be the alpha male who has the pick of sexual favours. They think I must be controlling the women, or they must be drugged or something. But it couldn't be more different. It's the girls who are the most sexual, with each other. I'm usually too tired to join in!' Dan insisted.

The women agreed with giggles. They were clearly keen

to paint themselves as a highly sexed bunch, regularly telling me about their sexual trysts and group orgies. Dan repeated his point about the girls being sexual with each other so many times that I couldn't help but question whether their sexual appetites stemmed from their own libidos or because they view liberal sexual attitudes as a non-conformist act of rebellion.

'Sometimes it gets really full-on in here. It's not uncommon for someone to start licking someone out here on the kitchen table while someone else is cooking,' said Amanda, one of the naked ones. They then started to drop in comments about their individual sexual preferences and eccentricities.

'Fran over there is probably the most sexual out of everyone,' said Rachel. 'She can bring herself to orgasm just by thinking about sex. Isn't that true, darl'?' She turned to Fran, who was still stuck like glue to Suzy. But Fran just nodded and continued to stare at me. She hadn't said a word all evening and didn't for the remainder of my stay. Instead, she fixated her eyes on me – huge, startled, suspicious eyes.

'Women are amazing,' Lillie inputted. 'We are all so different. When I came into this commune 10 years ago, it was a gorgeous learning process, getting to know what makes each person come. Some of us need rubbing, others licking. Some of us come very easily, for others it takes time.'

'We know ourselves much better than most women because with women you take more time and get to discover yourself,' said Rachel. 'Being sexual with women is a totally different experience than with men. It's about experiencing pleasure, not pleasing the man. I learned recently that I come very differently if someone rubs the left side of my clit to my right side of my clit. Women don't get to know these things with men.'

All the girls said they were bisexual except for Amanda and Rachel. They declared themselves strict lesbians and were legally married to each other and the only two who did not share the master bedroom.

The master bedroom! Yes, let me tell you about that. It was a huge room with five double mattresses on the floor, pushed up together on the back wall to form one big bed – a makeshift super-duper-double-emperor-king size that sleeps 13 in a row. There were three other double bedrooms: one was used as an office, another was where the lesbian couple, Amanda and Rachel, slept and the last one was what they called the 'privacy room', which is where they went for orgies.

(May I add at this point that the 'privacy room' was where I stayed – thank goodness for my thick, woolly pyjamas, which provided some degree of body shield – eugh!)

'We don't use the main bedroom for sex – sleep is too important! If one of us is horny, we will say, "I feel like a wank, does anyone want to join me?"' one of the mousy blondes clarified. It could have been Chrissie or Suzy. Maybe Bettina. I could only distinguish the naked ones, and Rachel, because she was funny. 'Sometimes one of us will follow, or sometimes we'll all descend there like mad, crazy, sex-starved animals!'

'The spare room is also where we go if we need some time on our own,' added another.

'But that rarely happens,' interjected Lillie. 'When monogamous couples say they want time on their own, it's usually because their partners aren't giving them the freedom to be themselves. We accept and love each other so deeply that we don't have that need.'

At that point Tania made her debut appearance. She opened the door slowly, ceremoniously, relishing its theatrical effect. 'Hello, my love. Are they looking after you?' she bellowed in her deep, husky, slow voice.

Tania was a big, powerful girl, who commanded attention. 'Oh, my back!' she wailed with an accompanying dramatic swipe to her forehead. She then proceeded to lie face down on the kitchen table, pointing out that frontways was the only position in which she could remain stationary. Thankfully the plates had already been cleared by Lillie. And there we stayed for the next three hours, sitting round the wooden table, discussing love and sex, with Tania lying face down in the middle of it like a sacrificial creature.

Tania brought a new energy to the evening, not least because all her contributions to the conversation were made with her nose in the woodwork, but she also brought humour and fresh insights. Some of her sentences were admittedly a little morphine laced, but still she had stories, made jokes and her presence encouraged the rest of the group to be more comfortable with me. After all, she was the one who had given the OK for my visit.

'We were just telling Helen that it's the women in this relationship who are the most sexual,' said Dan, returning once more to his favourite point.

'So true,' said Tania slowly, her voice muffled from her position. 'I've always been a raving nymphomaniac. I think my parents knew that I was sex mad from about age five when I discovered my fanny and started playing with it, whenever and wherever I could – shamelessly.

'I've easily slept with over 1,000 men. We used to be in a

band and we became known for being the band that would have sex with anyone who asked – fans, journalists, guys who couldn't get laid any other way. I love sex. I would love to spend four days straight in a blackened room filled with hundreds of naked bodies and indulge in a fest of pussy, cock, sperm, sweat – everything. Stagger out, have a drink and go back in again. I think a lot of people in this room would love that, but sadly with the HIV risk, you just can't do that any more.'

Any more?

'Do you use condoms with each other?' I asked, glad to have a pick-up point away from this conversation.

'Among us, no – because we have all been tested and we have an absolute rule that if we do have sex outside of the relationship, we use protection. That is the single most important rule. Breaking it would be unthinkable.'

Despite their wanton sexual appetites they lived a clean life. They didn't drink much, they have 'treats Friday', where they buy chocolates, wine and 'lots of lovely things' from the village deli, but the rest of the week they stay sober and go to bed at 10 p.m. They get up early. Four of the girls work as painters and decorators and have to be up at six, which means Lillie gets up at 5.30 a.m. to fix their breakfast. As we talked, there was no music, no TV, no wine, just our conversation and the warmth of the AGA.

I asked how a new person ends up joining the group and would they be open to even more people joining their *ménage à dix-sept.*

'Everyone has come into the relationship through a love affair,' answered Tania, who seemed to be the natural leader. She was older than the others and I noticed how they pandered to her, fussing over her bad back, offering her painkillers, massage and water. 'For instance, I fell in love with her.' She pointed to one of the naked ones – Isobel, I think. 'I just had this overwhelming want for her as soon as I lay eyes on her at a music festival. I brought her to meet this lot and they fell madly in love with her too!'

'How do you know that you're all in love?' I asked. 'Say, Isobel falls in love with Chrissie and Katie, but not with Dan and Amanda? Or say, you, Chrissie and Katie fell in love with the newcomer, but Amanda didn't?' It sounded as if I was reading a GCSE logic problem.

'If a new person is going to come into the house, we all have to approve. But usually we find that if one person feels something, then the others feel the same. We are very in tune with each other,' said Dan, before adding, 'It's strange, what you find when you live in a communal environment is that you start to think as a group and you stop thinking as one person. A few years ago when we were living in Andorra and decided to move to Scotland, it wasn't like we had a vote on whether to move; we all felt it at the same time. You stop thinking as one person.'

'Do you have favourites?' I asked Tania. 'When you fell in love with Isobel, would that mean you loved her more than others in the house for a while?'

Tania took a deep breath, her back and shoulders rising up from the table, where she was still lying face down, as if bracing herself for executing an explanation of this complicated concept. 'We all love each other very, very deeply but it isn't like we love each and every one of us at a constant level. At any one time we might fall for one particular person in a highly charged way. So at the moment I am just madly in love with this one here...' She raised her neck as high as she could, just enough to make eye contact with Katie, who smiled appreciatively and reached out an arm to affectionately touch Tania's hand.

'We call it flu,' Rachel chipped in. 'Because you can't control it, and it often puts you in bed!' They all laughed in agreement, proud of their *bon mot*.

'Those two over there have a serious case of it,' Dan added, referring to Fran and Suzy, who were still in an embrace and therefore completely mute. 'If someone starts following someone around, or if two of us start disappearing up to the privacy room a lot, we say: "They've got flu." But then they'll recover and they might become obsessed with someone else.'

I ask whether they experience jealousy when two of them get all feverish. 'I can't believe it's taken you this long to ask!' laughed Tania. 'Most people ask about jealousy straightaway, but if you truly love someone, you want them to be happy.'

'When monogamous couples get jealous because they see their partner talking to someone else, it comes from pure self-interest,' declared Dan. I noted how he self-styled himself as a psychology expert on a number of issues. 'They want their partner for themselves. But if I love someone, why would I not want them to have some fun with someone else?'

'We experience envy but sexual jealousy is a very different thing,' he continued. 'As a guy, if I was watching my girl get fucked and he had a great body, a perfect torso and was well endowed, then yes, I could get envious about that. But that is very different to feeling resentful that he is fucking my woman. It takes a decision to feel jealous.'

'We need a hell of a lot of honesty in this house,' admitted Tania. 'That's something which takes a bit of getting used to. We are open about our feelings and insecurities on a level most people can't comprehend. When something bugs us, we say so. We lay down every single thought that goes through our minds and we learn not to take things personally.'

'Men struggle with that more,' asserted Dan. 'Every problem we've ever had about jealousy or possession has been with men. They try to blame any tension in the house on women but it's usually men that create it. That's why we've seen more men come and go in this relationship.'

Their claim to selfless love stretched beyond sexual possessiveness to materialistic belongings too. 'All our income is pooled, like it would be with a couple,' Lillie explained. 'Our assets are shared. We love each other, why would we want to keep our possessions and wealth separate? Dan looks after the money. He's good at that sort of thing and we're happy for him to have the responsibility.'

They were obviously keen to convey that their group dynamic could easily operate like a couple dynamic, but it seemed to have escaped them that even the closest of couples can remain cautious when it comes to possessions. You would think, when there are 17 people with a share of the pot, they would be well within sanity to protect their individual assets. But surprisingly, perhaps worryingly, they all appeared content that their assets and income would be taken off their hands and managed by Dan.

'We don't ration each other. If someone wants to buy something, we say go and buy it, but as you can see, none of us in here trot around in Jimmy Choos!' quipped Rachel.

'If someone says they want 15 quid, I give them 15 quid and don't ask what it's for. But if someone says they want 500 quid, I might ask why,' explained Dan. 'When we go out, I manage the purse for all of us. It makes sense. Being the guy, I'm less likely to get my purse snatched.' Blimey, I thought, what sort of Scottish village is this, if a woman isn't safe carrying a purse?

'We don't have the need for possessions that most people do. We're a commune, we don't follow a consumer lifestyle,' explained one of the naked ones. 'We have some favourite things that are sacred to us. One of us might have a favourite top that we keep for ourselves. Kitty has hers on now.' At the sound of her name Kitty looked up from picking wood splinters out of the chair and did a proud little shimmy, puffing her chest out to show off her baby pink T-shirt. 'We don't ever clock things up. If we see something in a shop, or if we somehow come into possession of something, we'll be like: "Oh, so-and-so would love that. Give it to her!" We know what makes each of us happy.'

* * *

I did wonder just how much the women of this group cleaved to the polyamorous lifestyle of their own free will and how much was blind group conformity. Dan was overzealous in declaring that the commune was not male controlled but it was only the women who went out to work. It was he who controlled the finances; it was men who tended not to stick it out. All of the women were on the Pill. I'm not saying Dan crumbled them into Lillie's curries, but it struck me as odd that 16 women, most of fertile age, would choose to remain childfree and all concede to taking hormonal contraception, which many women find disagreeable.

Their happy family, supposedly oozing with love, care and affection for each other, came at a high price. They had effectively surrendered their identity to be part of it. In fact, the commune's dynamic epitomised everything about my reluctance to be in a relationship. When Dan said, as he was describing their decision to move to Scotland 10 years ago, 'You stop thinking for yourself after a while', the hairs on my neck stood up! I'm scared of becoming lost in the identity of one other person, let alone being lost in the identity of a group. Yet this group relished such a sense of group belonging.

These 16 women and one man had no time of their own and no opportunities to develop their own views or interests. As I've continually made clear throughout this book, all relationships require a certain degree of sacrifice so perhaps those who crave a relationship the most are the ones who find some sort of solace in entrusting a part of their self-identity to others. As Jake, the bachelor we met in Chapter One, said, 'It's more responsibility to be alone.' It is easy to blame under-achievements and shortcomings on the fact that we are tied to someone else. Jake described living with ex girlfriends as being 'low ambition'. Likewise, this group, sitting on wooden chairs around their apparent leader, tummy down on the dining table, sought no such satisfaction from realising ambitions. They lived day in, day out, sharing food, never wanting for anything in faded T-shirts, while having lots of sex, listening to music, thinking, talking, and for four of them, going out to plaster and paint walls.

For most of us our career, personal achievements, even our hobbies are definitive. These are what make me get up in the morning. When we introduce ourselves to someone new and say what we do, where we live or any other top line information, we are telling them, 'This is who I am, this is what I've done with my life', and most of us derive satisfaction from that. Our possessions are also a personal stamp. My clothes, my battered old books, my photos, my 56 pairs of shoes (I'm guessing, really), my research files stacked on my desk, my beady jewellery – these are all symbols of what is happening in my life. But this group had none of those things. Their values and goals could not be further away from mine. They seek refuge in group identity whereas I run away from it. If I'm a commitment-phobe, these were commitment *addicts*! Perhaps there is a correlation between those who seek to be consumed by a relationship and those who struggle to identify what they really stand for.

CHAPTER 10

Spreading the Love

In *No More Silly Love Songs*, author Anouchka Grose writes: 'You could see the whole of human history as a series of social experiments with the management of sexuality at the heart of each trial. So far, no group has managed to resolve the problem perfectly.'

In the Western world we have prescribed monogamy for our archetypical marriage. So indoctrinated is the one-man-one-woman template that anything else seems immoral, bohemian or even barbaric. But our fairytale template of fulfilling, monogamous love is not a well-trodden path. Monogamy was only cited in 20 per cent of the world's cultures according to the well-known anthropologist George Murdoch's classic *Atlas of World Cultures*, which listed and described every single known culture in the world and was last updated in 1981.

Even marriage itself cannot be easily defined. Anthropologists, historians and sociologists have been debating its common denominator but have yet to find one.

In some West African societies for example, a woman can be married to another woman but they won't have a sexual relationship. They will just team up for work and community duties. In parts of China, Japan and Sudan indigenous people can marry ghosts or spirits (it's a way of transferring wealth between families if there is no marriage suitor). If the Bella Coola and Kwakiutl native societies of the Pacific Northwest were really desperate to become in-laws one family could marry a child to another family's dog.

As we saw in Chapter Four, before modern civilisation, human societies organised themselves into large clans and sexual possession was an alien concept. Those values are still alive and well in tribal communities. Even so, they vary widely. In Amazonian societies such as the Araweté, the Mehinaku, the Tapirapé and the Wari, people believe in something known as 'partible paternity'. When women become pregnant, they are thought not to have completely conceived yet – they are just 'a bit pregnant'. To ensure the development of the foetus, the woman must continue to have sex with lots of men. It's believed that each man's sperm will add something to the development. The woman, naturally wanting the best traits for her child, will seek 'contributions' from the strongest, funniest, kindest and best-looking men in the village. This certainly does not augur well for monogamy but according to the anthropologist Christopher Ryan in *Sex at Dawn*, 'Instead of these men being blinded by jealousy, men in these societies find themselves bound to each other by shared paternity for the children they've fathered together.'

Until recently the Marind-anim people of Melanesia believed that a bride's fertility depended on her being filled with the semen of several men on her wedding night. Ten members of the groom's lineage would line up to have sex with her and similar rituals would be repeated throughout her married life because it was thought to help with fertility.

Among the Moso, an ancient society in southwest China, near to the border of Tibet, paternity is inconsequential because everyone appears to have sex with whomsoever they choose, non-possessively. They have no word for husband or wife but refer to them with the same word for friend. Marriages are temporary and don't involve the exchange of property, care of children or expectations of fidelity. Men and women may foster as many relationships, or *acia* as they are known, as they please and they can end them as they choose. They implicitly respect each other's autonomy. A request for fidelity would be interpreted as an attempt to negotiate an exchange of some sort.

The Moso are a matrilineal society – that means inheritance passes down the female line. Anthropologists have noted that in all matrilineal societies there tends to be a disregard for legitimacy of children. Sexual partners end up being non-exclusive and any resulting children are loved and cared for by all of the adults in the village – a practice known as allo-parenting or infant sharing.

Many of the communities mentioned above, as well as the Efe people in the Congo and the Lisu of Burma, consider allo-parenting normal. Just as the development of the foetus is down to the contributions of several men's sperm, the development of the child is attributed to the nursing of several women. Grandmothers and even friends will muck in on breastfeeding. Every woman who partakes is considered a mother. Children wander happily into all the houses in the village and every adult has a duty of parental care.

While the modern four-bedroom house of the polyamorous

commune in Scotland is far removed from the tribal shelters of the sexually liberated matrilineal societies of the undeveloped world, their willingness to surrender their independence and live as a group was similar. Perhaps the more communal a society, the more romantic and sexual intimacy it can handle. Conversely, perhaps the more independent a society becomes, the less consolidated sexual partners need to become.

There is actually an annual event for the romantically adventurous to discuss multi-loving in the modern world. It attracts the polyamorous-minded, but not those who seek the same intense relationships as the Scottish commune. Held every autumn in a community centre in the depths of the Devonshire countryside, the event is called OpenCon, after the better-known BiCon, a gathering for bisexuals. It's billed as a 'safe place for people to explore ethical non-monogamy'.

* * *

I can safely say the clientele at OpenCon 2012 was far removed from the crowd at the stately Halswell House. In place of the Bentleys and Porsches were caravans and battered old estates. Instead of my Agent Provocateur, this time I donned jeans, wellies and a warm duffle coat.

I arrived – shame on me – in a taxi, which I soon sensed was highly inappropriate for such a libertarian event. As the black Chevrolet with its bright yellow taxi sign crawled its way up the dirt track lined with tents, it cruised past bearded men in trench coats making their way to base camp. We passed four women, two of whom had pink hair. These people may be pioneers of an open sexual lifestyle but they certainly didn't think they needed Jimmy Choos to increase their chances!

Standing by the entrance to the old farmhouse were two women. One was wearing a bright coloured cotton summer dress, with clashing patterned tights, topped off with a fleece. The other wore a long dress with odd coloured stockings – not odd as in a strange colour but odd as in *different* colours – pink on the left leg and green on the right! There were lots of tie-dye fabrics and thick velvet skirts. Cardigans went over everything, including other cardigans.

I had arrived just in time for the introductory class – Poly 101 – aimed at polyamorous newbies. The veterans had gone off to more advanced workshops such as 'how to deal with jealousy', 'poly-parenting' or 'poly troubleshooting skill share'. Poly, I soon learned, is short for polyamorous – the act of loving more than one person at a time. Everyone bandied the word 'poly' around. Calling it polyamorous would be like saying mathematics instead of maths or mobile phone instead of phone.

Some poly people get very pedantic when it comes to the difference between being 'poly' and 'open'. For the sake of simplifying things, an open relationship is an umbrella term for lots of types of non-monogamous relationships; poly is one type within that definition, and swinging would be another.

Poly people celebrate love, not sex. They didn't strike me as being a particularly randy bunch, so I can understand why they get annoyed when the media mistakes them for being libidinous bed-hoppers. As one organiser said, 'People hear polyamory and they think we're swinging from chandeliers and having an orgy. In fact, a polyamorous group are more likely to be sitting and having a cup of tea.'

Sitting and drinking a cup of tea was exactly what the

people around me were doing now as we waited on the grass for the Poly 101 class to start. It had already been delayed by 20 minutes. I looked around to see who I could talk to and pounced on a shy-looking blonde in her early 30s. Tina was apparently here with her boyfriend, though he'd gone to a different class. It was the first time they'd attended the conference but they had been to several poly meet-up groups back in London, where they lived. 'I knew that I had a different attitude to relationships when I was a teenager. I remember my friend saying sorry because she'd kissed the same guy that I was dating – I think she was expecting some sort of drama, but I just said, "Brilliant, go for it!" I liked the idea we could share the same guy! It wasn't until I met my current partner 10 years later that I felt I had finally met someone who shared my views. The thing was we didn't know how to go about having the open relationship that we had always fantasised about. We went swinging a few times, but it wasn't us – it's a posey atmosphere. They don't really care who you are, it's nameless sex: we wanted more, we wanted actual relationships.'

I couldn't ask her too much. My visit to OpenCon was another undercover mission. As with my trip to the sperm donor mothers' group, I'd contacted the organisers to see if I could attend as a journalist for research but was greeted with silence. So I went ahead regardless. Since I was genuinely interested in exploring non-conventional relationships and meeting other love rebels like myself, I wasn't strictly a fraud but it did mean that I couldn't ask too many probing questions.

There were around 20 people in the Poly 101 class. Our instructors, Liz and Nick, looked about 12, but were in fact 22 and 26.

'Being poly to me is about rejecting the finite model of love,' Liz began, once the class introductions were out of the way. 'I don't believe love is a finite resource and spreading it amongst more than one person doesn't necessarily dilute it, so I see no reason to ration it, or deny it to people.'

Liz had two partners, one she saw nearly every day as he lived near her and the other once or twice a month, since he lived in a different city. She also had several occasional lovers. 'It's not that I get one thing from one person and a different quality from another and that's why I feel complete,' she clarified. 'All of them are complete relation-ships and they are unique individuals.'

Nick had been with his girlfriend for two years. With her consent, he also had a casual boyfriend, who was engaged to a girl who was dating one of his girlfriend's other boyfriends. Confused? Don't worry, it's not important. It was now Nick's turn to talk to the group.

'In Western culture the definitive way to express true love is through fidelity but for me that never made sense.' Short, baby-faced with huge spectacles, he spoke slowly, like a university lecturer, with his hands clasped in front of him. 'From a very early age the idea of pairing off with one person and only being with one person just seemed strange. Why can I only love one person and not others? Yet I can have a favourite book and love other books.

'I'd always felt like this but I didn't have a word for it. Even as a teenager when someone left me and started dating someone else, I never got angry like my friends did: I was simply happy for them. When I was 18, I was in a mono relationship with a girl but I had feelings for someone else. I googled something like 'can you love two people?' and that's how I came across poly relationships; I instantly related to it. I asked my girlfriend how she felt about exploring poly in the future. She said, 'That's not for me but if you want to do that, you should, on your own.' So I did.

'At first the process of adapting to poly relationships was difficult – you have to unlearn everything you've learnt about relationships. The idea that kissing someone else is wrong and immoral, for example. But I now see poly and mono as the equivalent of gay and straight: you either develop these feelings or you don't. My parents have been monogamous for 40 years so I know monogamy works, but it's just not for me. I develop feelings for other people when I'm still in love and I can't help that.'

Someone asked: 'What if you fall in love with one of your new partners and you're so crazy about them you don't want to spend time with your more serious partner?'

'It happens all the time!' Liz exclaimed. 'It's what we call "new relationship energy". You have to be careful at the start of a new relationship – you get a strong buzz so it's important to make time for your more established partner.'

I smiled at the term 'new relationship energy'. Now I knew it was the dopamine and norepinephrine of romantic love kicking in.

'But couldn't that buzz for someone new make you fall out of love with your usual partner and then you'd just resent spending time with them?' the class member insisted, clearly concerned.

'You can't put a quantity on love,' insisted Nick, who I later learned was a philosophy masters student and talked exactly like one. 'That doesn't make linguistic sense. What is a unit of love? It's an impossible question. I have a different quality of love for each of my partners but not a different quantity. I love my boyfriend but he is engaged and lives with someone else; that is very different to Kitty, who lives with me and whom I see every day. I give the people I see the same respect and consideration but I can't imagine how I could measure my love for them.'

Then Liz chipped in, 'I keep a public Google calendar so everyone I'm seeing knows when I'm free. Each of my partners has a colour so I can easily see if I've allocated enough days to them. I block some days out, too – that's important or you end up having no time for yourself.' There were gentle snorts of amusement around the room but Liz was not joking. Polyamory requires precision dating, planned with the same punctiliousness as a busy executive's diary.

There is something about romance that demands we be spontaneous about it. We don't expect to be keeping files, lists, records and calendars to keep track of the person we are head over heels in love with. But if you claim to be head over heels for five people, then practicality has to take over. In 2012 a banker called David Merkur gained online notoriety after his spreadsheet of his eight Internet dates went viral. There was a column for their interests, where they first met, how many dates they'd had, what he thought of them and how far he'd gone. He sent it to one of the women on his spreadsheet, thinking she would be flattered by how much she shone out compared to his lesser entries. But she didn't see it as such a compliment. Outraged, she hit 'forward' and Merkur's love chart went all around the world.

Personally, I don't blame him. I know from my own experiences that Internet dating gets confusing. Everyone you contact has a real name, a profile name and usually an email alias that doesn't correspond to either. Given the number of stop-start interests and date cancellations, you need to juggle at least 10 interested parties at a time. Without Excel, how else are you supposed to remember who's who? It won't be long before there are apps to manage and record notes on your dates. Now there's a *Dragons' Den* success in the making.

* * *

Nearly everyone I spoke to throughout my two-day stay at OpenCon reported some sort of lightning bolt moment when they at last identified as polyamorous. Their accounts were strikingly similar to what asexual individuals reported. People discussed their fears about 'coming out' as poly; they talked about their anguish at feeling 'different' until they discovered they were not alone in their multi-loving ways. Most said that the only reason they had agreed to monogamous relationships in their earlier years was because they thought they had to.

At lunch I shared a table with Carl, a 53-year-old academic. His face was gaunt with hollow cheekbones but underneath those wizened features I could see the bone structure of a once very attractive man. In a jacket and jeans, he was sartorially far superior to the typical OpenCon reveller with his/her imaginative charity shop ensemble. As a single male Carl had arrived with a female friend. As with the Eyes Wide Sin party, lone males were not permitted.

Carl had a 10-year-old son from a previous relationship. He was now in an open relationship with a woman who lived in Canada. 'We have a great relationship – we travel to places together a few times a year and stay with each other a couple of months but we both see other people,' he told me.

'I've always been in monogamous relationships but only by default,' he continued. 'I don't think I'm capable of enduring love, if I'm honest. I've always thought there should be more. My past partners always knew that I was keen to introduce another party to our sex life but none of them wanted to go there and I never wanted to throw a good relationship away for it. I've done a lot of sneaking around over the years; I look back and feel terrible guilt about how I deceived some of the women I was supposed to be true to. I didn't know that you could be honest about these things – I thought the only way to have sexual experiences with other people was to be dishonest about it.

'When I split up with my son's mother I tried swinging and even used websites to meet couples. I liked it at first because it was a novelty but I went right off it after a year.'

'Why?' I asked.

'It's sex on a plate. When sex comes easily there's nothing appealing about it. It's not so much the chase I want, but more the...' He paused to think of the right word. '...The build-up and the connection you have after sex. Courting is our human mating ritual.

'I met my current partner online six years ago and she suggested an open relationship. I knew at once that this was what I'd always wanted. I was filled with a sense of warmth that she understood; I relaxed. I'd always battled against my desires to see other people before but with her I didn't have to. I now think you get more closeness with open relationships – you know more about each others' lives than anyone else, but you don't have all the emotional obligations which so often lead to resentment. And anyway, usually I find that a fling elsewhere makes me appreciate how fantastic she is. I feel utterly fulfilled with the type of relationship I have now.'

Yet Carl couldn't share this new sense of fulfilment with peers and family. Stigma prevented him from doing so. 'My career would be ruined if I came out as poly,' he said sadly. 'I'd never advise anyone to confess they were open if they don't want to be ostracised.'

Celine, a 27-year-old bisexual library worker, knows that only too well. She had a serious girlfriend as well as several casual relationships with both men and women. 'People reacted so much worse to me saying I was open than they did to me admitting I was bisexual,' she told me. 'People at work were OK when I said I was bi – they were even interested in my love life! But when I told them I have open relationships, they were repulsed. Now at work I feel like I'm judged.'

Another woman, Jess – tall and slim, with short cropped black hair and a long, flowing dress – had brought her two-year-old son with her. She jumped at Celine's comment. 'We have to defend being open a lot,' Jess said, 'especially since we have children.' 'We' referred to Jess and her partner of three years. They lived together with their son and one of Jess's lovers, there temporarily. That wasn't unusual – her partner's lovers had also stayed for several weeks at a time. If you think that's complicated, Jess also had a 10-year-old daughter with a different man – also polyamorous. At weekends the daughter regularly stayed with her dad, who apparently lived in a house with three other polyamorous people.

'The first thing people say is, "What about your children?"' said Jess. 'It's not as if we're performing sex acts in front of them! My children get so much love. In fact, with polyamorous people, there is far less conflict between parents who are no longer together than mono couples who split up. My daughter's dad comes round all the time. If he wanted to come on holiday with me and my current partner, it wouldn't be a problem. People assume that we must be fraught with jealousy. I'm not saying our relationships are perfect or that we don't argue or have egos like everyone else but there's no possession or resentment which I see in so many traditional couple parents.'

* * *

Raising the respectability of polyamory is one of the aims of OpenCon and an ongoing mission for the community. Active members have started a group called Polytical, which campaigns for recognition of multiple relationships within the counselling and health professions. It also campaigns against what it calls 'poly-discriminatory' laws. For example, it wants to stamp out regulations requiring rented houses with more than five people to have licences. Polytical says these laws make it hard for a relationship of more than five people to live together; also it's unfair that paternity laws only recognise one parent. These campaigns may sound ludicrous to us now, but perhaps one day we will see a parliamentary Bill to allow multiple marriages just as we have for same-sex marriages.

As Nick, the philosophy student, said, 'There are people from all walks of life who are poly, including solicitors and bankers, but when it comes to 'coming out' it tends only to be people in creative professions – artists and writers or those in IT, where convention doesn't always apply. That's why poly people are viewed as a bit quirky. Most people have no problem with sexual non-monogamy but it's the idea that you can *love* two people that they find most weird.'

The main problem poly people face when it comes to being integrated into respectable society is that they tend to be insular. And it's easy to see why: they have no time to go out with non-poly friends because they're always out with dates. As one young guy observed: 'It helps if the people you are dating are dating your partners' friends.' Sound advice for time management, but it means that poly people only ever mix with other poly people and the result is a small clique where everyone knows everyone. This could explain why many of them seem to harbour a defiant mono-people-don't-understand-us attitude and could also explain the rebellious undertones in their choice of clothes and shocking pink striped stockings.

I certainly saw this in-crowd exclusivity among the established OpenCon attendees. It seemed to be either you're in the poly club, know the lingo, have dyed your hair a psychedelic colour and have dated all the important people. Or you're a newcomer, can't control 'new relationship energy' and are still struggling to comprehend feelings of jealousy like a mere mono person.

Liz revealed a little of this psyche during our Poly 101 Class: 'I love it when you're at an event with lots of different partners. Someone who's not on the poly scene sees you with one of your partners, then later they see that person with their arm around someone else. They look ever so confused,' she grinned, proud and pleased to have left all those boring monogamous sheep perplexed.

As is often the case with insular communities, they create their own lexicon. There is a whole host of labels for concepts that the hetero-monogamous couple would never need. A 'metamore', for instance, is your partner's partner, while a 'sweetie' is a casual sexual partner. There are triads (three-way relationships) or quads (four-ways). Your personalised network of partners plus their partners and their partners' partners needs to be mapped out using tree diagrams and so there is a delightful term for that too: polycules! As one girl pointed out in a discussion workshop, 'Just because you're in an open relationship doesn't mean you can't cheat.' However, I found it ironic that polyamorous people delight in swaying from convention yet their relationships are governed by rules – lots and lots of highly complex and painfully brokered rules tailored for each couple, triad or quad. It seemed to me that if the rules aren't individualised enough, there's less approval in the poly clique because the relationship could be seen as too standard.

The variations are endless. Some poly circles are open (if everyone you are dating is open to date anyone). Some are closed (if everyone you are dating agrees that they can only sleep with *specific* people). Some poly people hierarchise their partners, nominating a 'primary' partner as the one they share most of their life with and everyone else as 'secondary'. Others love and cherish each person they are involved with equally. Some couples only allow their partner to date someone of the same sex; some of the more possessive poly types only allow their partner to date someone in a primary relationship, presumably because a loved-up paramour won't pose such a threat as an emotionally available one.

Monogamous relationships have rules, of course but they are mostly universal and unspoken. The writer Meg Barker makes this observation in her relationship self-help book *Rewriting the Rules*: 'People in monogamous relationships assume they have a shared set of rules when in fact they don't,' she told me when I asked her about the golden rules of open relationships. 'One might think it's OK to go online and look at porn but the other might be horrified; one might think it's OK to stay friends with an ex, but the other might be hurt by that. In open relationships people bring all these things up and negotiate from the start.'

I have to say this was not selling the idea of an open relationship to me. When last in a proper relationship I found it bothersome enough dealing with drawing up the rules as to who drives home from a party. If I had *five* fully integrated relationships to draw up boundaries and ground rules for, my life would be one big boardroom discussion. A woman in every port may be a good idea if the other women in the other ports don't get involved with each other, but if they've all got to sign up to a mutual treaty, that's one serious diplomatic operation.

As my stay at OpenCon was coming to an end, I came across a couple who clearly hadn't had any rule-setting discussions when they got together. The result was really very sad. As I took a seat in the canteen on my last evening, I met Alana. I put my plate of lentil stew and vegan coleslaw and bowl of chocolate and beetroot cake on the table next to a pretty brunette with glasses, looking very serious. I smiled and asked if she had enjoyed herself over the weekend.

'It was interesting,' she said abruptly with a strong accent. She was Polish and her husband German; they had been married and living in Frankfurt for a year. She pointed to him across the room, where he was munching away happily with another group of people, seemingly oblivious to her.

'Is it your first time here?' I asked.

'For me, yes; for him, no. I am definitely monogamous,' she asserted defiantly. She wouldn't know that I was there in a research capacity so she obviously presumed that I too was in the poly clique and her statement was an intentional barrier.

'What did you think of it?' I asked, ignoring her frostiness.

'I'm here to try to understand it,' she said, softening slightly. 'My husband is into this. After we married, he tells me that he is a member of this poly group – it was the first I heard. What can I do? We are married already. I either accept and try to understand this world he wants, or we split up and I go back to my country.'

Had she talked for one sentence more I was certain her voice would have shaken. She stared down at her plate, as if eye contact would have been too much. I wished I could offer some words of comfort. It was all right for me – I was here for research, high on the fascinating stories I had gathered – but I knew that in 12 hours' time I'd have a warm, dry minicab to take me to a waiting train, which would take me back to the sanity and solitude of my home. There I could resume dating who and when and how I liked. I wouldn't have my husband's difference of views overshadowing my day and making my eyes well up at the dinner table in front of a stranger. Polyamory was supposed to have been borne out of the ideals of free love yet Alana's marital set-up couldn't have been further from this. For her it was a prison of torment. That is perhaps why most of us are happy to adhere to a mainstream relationship model. If monogamy is de rigueur, it makes things safer for those of us like Alana, who just want a good old no-frills sturdy marriage. Generic rules are reliable. When the rules allow for a more gung-ho unrestrained set of values it can be quite a threat.

CHAPTER 11

Multi-cultural Mistresses

Despite these fascinating ways of conducting simultaneous relationships in tribal societies, and among the polyamorous community in the UK, throughout human history one of the most universal forms of marriage has been that between one man and several women. Or more formally: polygyny (not to be confused with polygamy, the umbrella term for a variety of multiple marriages). Polygyny has been socially acceptable in the majority of cultures at some point. However, the majority of marriages in these cultures have been monogamous – hardly surprising because the gender ratio simply wouldn't add up. But as an ideal, polygyny is a popular one.

Many of the Old Testament Prophets and Patriarchs had multiple wives, including Abraham, Jacob, Gideon, Saul, David, Solomon and more. Some interpreters claim even Moses had a second wife. Polygyny is still prominent today in many parts of the world. In Africa, having more than one wife signifies wealth and a man will have as many wives as he can afford. The number of children becomes his status symbol. This might sound expensive, but multiple wives is considered an investment because it will hopefully lead to more children, which will in turn raise the future earning capacity of the family clan. South African president Jacob Zuma is a fan of polygyny – at the time of writing he has four current wives and a couple of exes.

It's also alive and well in parts of South Asia including Thailand and rural China, even though officially it's been outlawed. Polygamy is permitted in Islam but in reality few practice it and some Muslim countries have even outlawed it. Closer to home, the Marquess of Bath, Alexander Thynn, is a well known preacher and practitioner of polygyny. He frequently appears in the press, no doubt because his aristocratic background and respectable vocations as politician and author are an unlikely backdrop to such an eccentric relationship lifestyle. The Marquess claims to have had more than 70 lovers since his marriage to the former actress Anna Gael Gyarmathy and has installed many of the women in cottages on his estate, referring to them as his 'wifelets'. He described his idealism once to *The Telegraph* thus: "My parents were monogamists and serial adulterers. They cheated on their ideal. Seeing their example, I preferred to have a different ideal, one I wouldn't cheat on. And my childhood fantasy – swimming along with a string of girls – suggests to me that, regardless of my parents, I inclined towards polygyny from a very early age.'

Polygyny's little sister is polyandry, where a woman has more than one husband. This is far rarer and, sorry to ruin any eroticised fantasy of a powerful Cleopatra-type being served by a harem of men whom she can pick and choose at her leisure, the reality of polyandry is far from this.

Polyandry is more symbolic of sexual slavery than matriarchal values. Most instances are fraternal polyandry, where one woman becomes the property of her husband's brothers and other relatives because they can't find their own wives.

Polyandry has been witnessed in Tibet, India, Bhutan, northern parts of Nepal, Nigeria, Kenya, the Nymba, Tanzania and some pre-contact Polynesian societies. Generally it was adopted in areas with poor farming conditions because landowners couldn't afford to distribute their holdings to all of their sons, so they encouraged them to share a wife. It also emerged in nations with a history of son preference and where female babies were left to die resulting in a male dominated population.

It may seem like polygyny (one man, several woman, in case you forgot) is far removed from 'wholesome' Christian societies but if you look at the many platforms that men have used to pursue multiple female lovers, you will see just how perennial a relationship model this is. Mistresses, paramours, courtesans, concubines, geisha and all manner of kept women have featured throughout history in all cultures and takes on almost as many forms today. Rather than saying that polygyny is the most practised relationship dynamic, I'd be more specific and say that the most common pattern is 'one man, one wife and one ancillary lover'.

The multimillionaire Sir James Goldsmith, who died surrounded by his mistresses, very famously said as much: 'When a man marries his mistress he creates an automatic job vacancy.' Some 1,700 years before him, Augustine of Hippo, a scholar of the Roman Catholic Church, recommended that men be granted the right to have concubines otherwise 'they would be driven to seduce other men's wives.' A few hundred years before him the great

Greek orator Demosthenes reputedly said, 'We have mistresses for pleasure, concubines to care for our daily body's needs and wives to bear us legitimate children and to be faithful guardians of our households.'

The ancillary lover is ubiquitous and her role is multifaceted. Historian Elizabeth Abbott provides lively accounts of all her many forms in *Mistresses: The History of the Other Woman*. In Imperial China, for instance, as far back as 221 BC noblemen and royalty had concubines, whole harems of them if they could, and continued to do so right up until the fall of the Qing Dynasty in 1912. Concubines were not shrouded in secrecy and shame as a modern mistress might be, but were an integral part of marriage. They had their domestic duties and legal rights spelt out. Far from a concubine being viewed as a lowly prostitute, she was a revered figure with a significant but distinct role to a wife. By law concubines were protected from potentially jealous scheming wives and similarly, a wife was protected from neglect by her husband, should he become too enamoured of his concubine. Very often they all lived under the same roof and the concubine could be expected to bear children for her master.

Sometimes concubines were even given as gifts to bridegrooms or businessmen. Imagine putting such a thing on your wedding list today! Unlike a wife, a concubine's social class didn't matter but her physical appearance most certainly did. So much so that she would be inspected and selected at a *mooi jais* – a concubine market. Men or someone acting on behalf of the man would inspect her feet and even sniff her nether regions – the sweeter the better, apparently.

In ancient Greece, wealthy men entertained *hatarea* – high-class, educated, cultural women, who traded sex for luxurious gifts and money. Considered more cultured and better educated than the average Attic woman, they were usually foreigners or former slaves, but in becoming a *hatarea* their income would afford them more freedom than a married woman of ancient Greece.

On the Indian subcontinent the 'other woman' took the form of a *tawaif*, also known as *Kanjri*. They entertained the nobility of the Muslim Mughal Empire during the sixteenth, seventeenth and eighteenth centuries. *Tawaifs* excelled and contributed to music, dance, theatre, film and the Urdu literary world. The popular ones would sometimes exert influence over the politics of the empire.

In France, in the nineteenth century a woman who was kept by her male lover was called a *lorette*, so named after the Notre Dame de Lorette church in Paris because it housed men of means who could afford to keep mistresses. The surrounding neighbourhood housed many such women, who would go to the church to visit their lovers. The writer Nicholas Green wrote fondly of the *lorette* in *The Spectacle of Nature*: 'Always elegantly dressed, the *lorette* peeps out coyly from a theatre box, engages in double entendre with male admirers at a masked ball, displays herself while enjoying the view from her apartment window. In a sense, for men she was quintessentially public property – to be discussed, admired, acquired...'

In Shia Islam there is the *sigheh*, a legal temporary marriage. This allows a man to get around the ban on sex outside of marriage. Originally, the *sigheh* was introduced by pre-Islamic Arabs for men who had to travel away from home for long periods of time, or were unable to commit fully to marriage. But he has to pay the woman for obliging, of course.

Even popes of the Catholic Church have a history thick with mistresses. In fact, the era from the ninth to the mid-eleventh century has been nicknamed 'pornocracy' because papal mistresses were so influential. Pope Agapetus produced a bastard son and this after knowing that he himself was the bastard son of a priest. And Pope John XIII was murdered by the jealous husband of one of his mistresses.[18]

The most intricate and expensive of the ancillary lovers is, as you may have already guessed, the Japanese geisha. A geisha is never expected to sleep with her clients; she just teases. Her appeal is that she represents a very different role from a wife. The ideal geisha is skilful, playful, carefree and flamboyant, while the ideal Japanese wife is modest, sombre and responsible. The geisha can dance, recite verse, play musical instruments and knows how to make every man feel like a million yen.

A geisha's lifestyle and training was usually funded by a patron called a danna san. I used to live in Japan and have a degree in the language. When I became enlightened to the culture of sugar daddy dating I couldn't help thinking that a 'sugar daddy' was much like a danna san. Typically a wealthy man, he was sometimes married, with the means to fund a geisha's education and expenses. Like a sugar daddy, he would most likely enjoy regular companionship and intimacy with his geisha but intimacy wouldn't be expected. He might well fall in love with her, but even so, he'd always go home to his wife and the relationship was not expected to last forever.

Mistressdom was also deeply entrenched in Royal Courts of Europe. The King would acquire a new lover, girlfriend

---

18 *Mistresses: A History of the Other Woman.* Elizabeth Abbott, Overlook Press, USA, 2011

or prostitute whenever he pleased to satisfy lusty desire or simply a whim. Sometimes his mistress would be married off to someone else to diffuse rumours, should she fall pregnant. France introduced a semi-official title for the monarch's other woman: the *maîtresse-en-titre* (mistress-in-chief). It was introduced as a direct result of King Henry IV's many lady friends during the sixteenth century. Whichever one was lucky enough to be appointed *maîtresse-en-titre* would secure herself a luxurious palatial apartment and a healthy allowance.

If smart, she could also command significant political influence in the courts. One official mistress who engineered things spectacularly well was Madame de Pompadour. Once she had won the heart of Louis XV, he granted her powers to determine all sorts of policy issues from military matters to foreign affairs to planning buildings. Pompadour didn't just look pretty and open her legs, she entertained her royal master with games of cards and read his daily reports for him. Poor health meant she wasn't always the raunchy, agile, enthusiastic bed-companion that the King might have hoped for so she made up for it with other enchanting female charms. The irony is that Madame de Pompadour had all the qualities a man now expects in a wife, but the relationship was meant to be short-term. Louis XV was probably no different in his sentiments to Jason, whom we met in Chapter Two. Jason said that he loved his wife because 'she made his life easier'.

English monarchs were just as amorous as the French. Henry II was particularly notorious for infidelities. So passionate were his feelings for one of his much younger mistresses, Rosamund Clifford, that his jealous wife plotted to kill her.

Charles II kept up his bed-hopping privileges throughout the Great Fire of London and the Great Plague in the seventeenth century. This obviously didn't go down well with his public and they called him the 'great enemy of chastity and marriage'. But at least he was decent to his mistresses, awarding them all titles and allowances, which went against the custom of the time, and elevated some of his illegitimate children to dukedoms. Five of today's 26 dukes are said to be the descendants of his love children.[19]

Charles II's most famous and longest serving mistress was Nell Gwyn, dubbed 'pretty, witty Nell' by Samuel Pepys for her quick humour. It's a remarkable rags-to-riches story, which has been made into a film several times over. Nell initially asked the King for £500 a year to be his mistress but was rejected as being too expensive. Instead she became his long-term mistress and continued to receive a Royal allowance even after his death.

Then there was King George IV, who had many public affairs. He offered his first mistress, Mary Robinson, £20,000 to take up the role but tired of her after a year and ended the affair without paying her. Penniless, she went to a newspaper and threatened to sell his love letters. He succumbed and agreed to pay her a small pension. *Plus ça change*!

Lorettes, courtesans, concubines, Royal mistresses and geishas are all variations of the ubiquitous role of an entertaining lover. Sought not for stability but as a muse, she offers more refined company to men than a prostitute, yet requires far less investment than a wife.

---

19 *Mistresses: A History of the Other Woman*, Elizabeth Abbott. Overlook Press, USA, 2011

MULTI-CULTURAL MISTRESSES

* * *

This milieu, I am afraid to say, is no different today. As Elizabeth Abbot concludes in *Mistresses*: "It is depressingly remarkable how the experiences of so many modern mistresses resemble those of mistresses past. Mistressdom remains an extension of marriage, a sanctioned outlet for male sexuality." I concur. When I was given the glamorous commission to go undercover on a marital affair website, the men I met all aspired to the same sense of duality in their love lives as had the historical male figures mentioned above. The first one, Justin, 45, good-looking, had a wife and three children back in his idyllic family home in the French countryside but stayed in London for business at least three days of the week. He too obviously felt there was a vacancy for a mistress – 'London can't give me everything,' he said. 'When I'm in France I do a different set of things – I'm a dad, I'm a gardener. When I'm here, I'm a professional and I have the bachelor lifestyle and I want someone to share that with – I like the fact I can switch.'

Trying not to sound too much like a journalist I asked if he could ever live either of these lifestyles exclusively. 'No,' he replied assuredly. 'I need the contrast. I could start a business in France and live the village life and be a doting husband, but that's not who I am. Or I could have the London lifestyle all the time but I need to go back to roots. I always look forward to going back to my wife and children – I need a place with familiarity.'

A Swiss businessman, who frequented the UK regularly, justified joining a cheating website by his mundane home life: 'It's all family, family, family – every day, your whole life! Everyone needs a bit of something outside of that.' He was currently on his second wife and had children with both women but the pressure of dedicating his whole life to either of them had clearly proved too much – 'You only have one life,' he said.

This man provided me with another insight into the adulterous predilections of the modern male. He had businesses in Romania and Bulgaria and looked after a team of 30 male labourers. Every six months he would pay for the all-male entourage to have a works-jolly in London. He expensed their flights, hotels and flash clubs and provided limousines and girls. Yes, girls. His workers had a typically Roman strong sense of family values. They were all married and doted on their wives back home but twice a year they considered it a rite of passage to get blindly drunk in a foreign country, sleep with escorts and visit strip clubs – all with the blessing of their Swiss employer.

Greg was another self-confessed philanderer who shared his story with me over email this time. As a 50-year-old successful freelance consultant, he had had several affairs throughout his 20-year marriage. 'I'm a walkabout,' he said. 'I get my energy and inspiration from being outside of the home unit so I've always found a reason to spend time away, but then I always wanted to go back.

'My wife is wonderful – she's allowed me to go off alone and get my energy and inspiration from outside of the home. She's never really complained about my projects, which take me away all the time. But that's because I've always come back more interesting than when I went. The only time things have ever been hostile is when I came home and I wanted to carry on living in my non-family mode. As long as I come back as the husband and father, I'm welcomed.'

Finally there was Mike, a slim fair-headed TV producer in

his early 40s. He enjoyed having 'a stable support network at home' but all romantic frisson between himself and his wife had gone.

'Before I married, I was a strong-minded, independent person with lots of interests. I played sport and would go away every weekend to visit friends in different places. One day a year ago I looked at this person in the mirror and thought, what happened to you?

'I felt hemmed in. All my decisions were influenced by the fact that I was married. There was a duality about my life – old me and the married me under the influence of my wife. I felt that I always did better at things when I was old me.

'I told my wife how I felt. I felt I was in danger of with-drawing from her if I didn't. But she was totally unreceptive and she said, "You need to grow up – that's pathetic!" That made it worse – you can't be yourself if you feel oppressed. I tried telling her again and she said I should go to counselling. But she wouldn't come with me because she said there was nothing wrong with our relationship – it was just my issue.

'Counselling was great, in retrospect. It made me take control of my feelings – I revisited the death of my parents and all sorts of things. I came out a more controlled, rational person but it didn't solve how I felt about my home life.'

During Mike's counselling programme, he almost became involved with someone at work but managed to stop himself. But the frisson of the flirtation and attraction put the idea in his head to have a fleeting romance with someone safer, outside his place of employment. And that's why he joined a website for married people looking for affairs.

'It's me seeking my old identity,' he mused. 'You compromise a lot in a marriage. If you like your space and your free time, it's a big ask to give that up. When I met my wife for the first four years we were infatuated. You lose control of reality when you fall in love. It's amazing but it isn't reality. It doesn't stay like that for a long time; it develops into something else but it will never be the same as it was at the beginning.'

'What does it develop into?' I asked.

'Friendship, really – I kept trying to notice things that would take me back to how I felt in the early days. I tried to remember why I had felt so strongly about her. You need admiration to feel like that again, but with such strong familiarity it's hard to feel admiration. It had become all about the kids. I felt I was secondary, mopping up the dregs of childcare. Every time I tried to tell her how I felt, she'd say the same things, "Grow up!" or "You can't live a student life forever!"'

Although I didn't approve of Mike's dishonesty in using such a website, I sympathised with his position. We are quick to condemn adulterers but as his case clearly showed, it was the overexpectations of unity that go with contemporary relationships that had driven him there. It is as if we view marriage as a parallel society, where we have to behave with a level of maturity as never before; as if marriage renders playful adventures and even individualism a thing of the past. It belittles anything that went before it as mere pre-marriage juvenility. Mike's affair was the only way he could think of to claw back his wilting self-identity.

I observed a consistent pattern with these men. They all had families and children removed from their fast-paced city professional lives, but they wanted to dip into bachelor life and find a low-maintenance lover to share it with. I never came across any man who expressed guilt about having a mistress; it was as if they felt it were an entitlement.

Today there are few things short of murder and child abduction as contemptible as adultery but in the past, particularly in the Middle Ages, extramarital love was considered a higher form of love than marital love. The Countess of Champagne once said that true love could not exist among people you were married to; the most daring and cool lotharios expressed their love outside of marriage. In the sixteenth century the essayist Montaigne wrote that any man in love with his wife was 'a man so dull no one else could love him'. The philosopher Seneca wrote that nothing is more impure than to love one's wife as if she were a mistress. It wasn't just the upper classes either. Many of the songs and stories told and sang by the lower classes derided marital love. It was dull and it was just plain weird.

The modern world still makes provisions for this philosophy. In France there is the *cinque au sept* – the two-hour window dedicated to clandestine encounters before each party goes home to their spouse. In Japan, where arranged marriages are still practised in some families, there are special 'love hotels' hiring out rooms by the hour. They are typically located on highways. No one works on reception, so guilty lovers can buy their room key discretely from a vending machine. I know – I've been to one! In the car park, very considerately, there are curtains around each parking space lest your car is recognised by your spouse (who is probably there with his/her own lover).

Our moralising climate may not like it but it is futile to try and quash the role of the ancillary lover. She is so deeply rooted in human history that it is hard to ignore her significance in the natural evolution of relationships.

* * *

As you can see, the extramarital female lover features most prominently among the wealthy classes and nobility. If a man has the means to keep an extra woman, he does so. One only has to take a snapshot of recent high-profile adulterers to get an idea of the temptation that wealth and power yields. Tiger Woods, Ray Parlour, General Petraeus, John Prescott, John Major, Jude Law, Arnold Swarzenegger, US presidential hopeful John Edwards, Bill Clinton, JFK and Berlusconi all had much to lose by being caught out by their illicit encounters, yet the risk didn't stop them.

On face value, it seems grossly unfair that it is men who get to have the best of both worlds. I know many a woman who would jump at the chance of dipping in and out of her marital role according to what other lovers are on the scene, but unfortunately the biological burden of childrearing and the psychological hold of her child always prevents her. But there is an upside: the reason why women the world over are willing to go along with this prevalent model of one man and multiple women is because, mostly, there's something in it for her too.

Historical examples abound of women using their role as muse to powerful men to their advantage. During the Ottoman Empire (roughly where modern Turkey is today), sultans kept scores of women in large *seraglios* (a harem). If one of the concubines was lucky enough to bear the Sultan a child, there was a good chance she would rise in rank to a

Gözde (The Lucky) an *Ikbal* (The Favourite) and receive luxury goods and her own servants.

In ancient Greece there was a young and beautiful woman called Aspasia. She could never be accepted into Greek society because she was a low-life foreigner, but using her beauty, charm and intelligence she managed to capture the heart of an influential Athenian statesman, Pericles. He wasn't that handsome himself but that didn't bother Aspasia. She won his adoration and soon her status as his lover allowed her to be accepted into society, and eventually made her a powerful figure in Greek society.

Even the media-dubbed 'professional mistresses' stir intrigue and fascination just as much as they evoke disapproval. Christine Keeler brought down a government but we remain captivated by her. In the 1960s, Vicki Morgan was nicknamed 'the beautiful bad girl' due to her love affairs with Alfred Bloomingdale, heir to the New York department store fortune, and actor Cary Grant. And who doesn't find the man manipulator Holly Golightly in *Breakfast at Tiffany's* simply adorable?

It's not just mistresses and muses. I often hear remarks from friends and colleagues laced with envy at other women's success in finding a well-established partner – 'She's bagged a banker', 'She married a doctor? She's done well'. No one ever expresses the merits of wealth outright but they don't exactly hide their approval either. Every time I tell my sister that I've got a date, she gets all excited but never forgets to ask whether 'he has a good job'. The partners of men with status often become publicly adored themselves – Princess Diana and The Duchess of Cambridge spring to mind.

There's a formal word for this status climbing. No, it's not gold digging, it's hypergamy – the practice of marrying up the social ladder. Anthropologically, hypergamy emerged in societies with little gender equality. Women would 'marry-up' to maximise their status and benefit their offspring while men would 'marry-down' socially, typically to a better-looking female. This is a classic exchange of beauty and youth for money and status, the result of which is still equality of power.

Today, you might just call it the WAG culture.

* * *

May I seize the opportunity to introduce the evolutionary theory of sexual selection? It sounds complicated but it's very simple and it says a lot about the dynamics of what men and women look to get from each other.

Darwin, and his protégés who have followed, deduced that a woman's fertility is more finite and more delicate than that of a male. Men are fertile for longer (*Playboy*'s Hugh Hefner fired fertile rounds at 74) and they can also sow their genetic seeds free from the burdens of pregnancy, child labour and child-rearing duties. Therefore a man can produce far more offspring than a female ever can. Over thousands of years, this gender injustice made women evolve to be far pickier than men. Well, if she's going to have to go through pregnancy, childbirth and feeding every time she has sex, she's sure going to pick a good one! This means men must compete for the female seal of approval. As the Natural History Museum put it on a big sign during its 'Sexy Beast' exhibition of 2011 about different species' mating strategies: 'Some battle it out with violent duels, others resort to dirty tricks. Females have the casting vote.

It's a female's prerogative to be demanding when choosing a mate'.

Sexual selection explains why women often flaunt their good looks to get ahead and men flaunt their faculty to provide. A woman's fertility was judged by primal man on how healthy and young she looked, but the indicator as to whether a male could produce healthy offspring was based on his ability to provide once the offspring were born, which is why attraction is judged on so very different parameters between the sexes. (Apply this next time a man makes a mocking comment about women and their silly shoes. Just remind him that it's a far cheaper posturing strategy than the male equivalent of buying silly sports cars.)

This is pretty much the established formula for the attraction between high-ranking men and their many forms of extra marital lovers. Many women don't need the intricate training of a geisha to play sexual selection to their advantage. In 2012, Channel 4 aired a reality documentary called *Rinsing Guys*. The 'rinser', the narrator told us, is a new breed of woman who has apparently mastered the art of persuading men whom they have never met to send gifts and money. The women had no intention of ever dating the men they flirted with online, but they knew just how to tease and charm them enough into sending gifts and in some cases, money. It's hard to know which is more abhorrent. The women for being so ruthlessly exploitative or the men for being so stupid!

I don't wish to sound like an outmoded antifeminist from the Victorian age, but sexual selection also explains why women don't jump so keenly into the sack for no-strings frolics as men do. We have seen how, when there is a shortage of women, societies adopt polyandry and share the women. The reverse is not the case, for women can tolerate celibacy far more easily. Also, in female prisons, there is little evidence of women becoming sexual with each other but in male prisons sexual favours and sexual abuse are well documented. There is also little evidence to suggest that in polygynous societies (where one man has multiple women) the girls become sexual with each other. While stories may abound in literature of bored concubines turning to lesbianism due to a lack of constant male attention, this is likely to be a myth playing to male fantasy rather than founded on historical evidence.

I will let you into another secret. During those youthful, dubious days of sugar-daddy dating, I learned only too well how women regularly play to the lesbian fantasies of men. One of my regular gentleman friends, whom I met every three months or so, would take me to dinner and then, after the second bottle of wine, insist we visit a private hostess club on Piccadilly called Churchill's. There, he'd blow thousands of pounds, requesting we have a drink with each one of the available girls so that I could pick my favourite, who we could take back to our hotel. Yes, *me* pick! Convinced that I loved it, he thought he was providing me with a great treat. How he ever got the idea that I would like to be pleasured by a woman into his head, I do not know – I had never expressed this. But actually it was him who got the thrill from it.

I was in the height of my sexual adventurousness at the time and doing such a thing had novelty value so I went along with it. But always, without fail, whatever happened between the girl and me was fake. The most interesting thing is that we didn't even have to confer that we would pretend, it was a given. Whoever the girl was, I let her lead the way because frankly I had no idea what I was supposed to be doing! She would let her hair drop in front of my face and pretend to kiss me. She'd put her hand under my groin and pretend to penetrate me. In reality she wouldn't even be touching. The idea that all women have secret Sapphic desires is nothing more than wishful male thinking.

That isn't to say that women don't enjoy sex or they only do it to entertain the predilections of men. But women's sex drives are more temperamental. A woman's sex drive needs nurturing; men's simply need igniting. Or, as the comedian Jerry Seinfeld put it: 'Men are like firemen. To men, sex is an emergency, and no matter what we're doing, we can be ready in two minutes. Women, on the other hand, are like fire. They're very exciting, but the conditions have to be exactly right for it to occur.'

The most alluring thing about the ancillary lover is that they are – my favourite phrase again – low-maintenance. They represent something more exciting than the sturdiness of a wife. Because marriage is no longer essential, there is now a growing number of men who want the mistress figure – a part-time lover at his beck and call – but they don't need to shroud it in secrecy because there is no wife. Most likely he does this because he's too busy doing other things to meet the taxing demands of a conventional relationship. If that's the case, he'll probably be expected to bring something else to the table, though. Otherwise what's it in for her?

Well, I bring you the mutually beneficial arrangement.

CHAPTER 12

Mutually Beneficial Arrangements

A typical profile on the dating site SeekingArrangment.com reads: '*Having worked hard for 15 years, I now want to spend more time enjoying myself. I'm looking for a fun female who knows how to party and enjoy life, who has a positive outlook and enjoys new adventures. An understanding of the demands of an entrepreneur when business deals are on is a must! From my side, I am willing to provide prudent financial support to the right woman to make a start in life, whether for her education or to develop a business.*'

Another one states: '*I am looking for a travel companion for a few weeks every year or until we tire of each other. I want a friendship but do not want a relationship that emulates marriage. I prefer an affectionate fun woman, educated, informed and with a sense of humour, a woman who is comfortable and happy with herself and her sexuality. I will obviously fund all mutual travel and make sure my lady has the means to turn herself out well for any occasion.*'

MUTUALLY BENEFICIAL ARRANGEMENTS

The women make it clear in their profiles that they're on the same page with these so-called 'arrangements': *'I'm educated, well travelled, attractive and laid-back and want to find the right guy to provide sparkling company for evenings out, weekends away, business engagements, whatever. In return I'd just expect respect, discretion and a little help in staying groomed, manicured and well-heeled!'*

Some are subtler: *'I am a classy, well-educated and well-travelled girl. I am attractive and graceful, diplomatic and sociable, adventurous and open-minded. I'm looking for an established man with old fashioned values who knows how to treat a lady and can take care of me.'*

The website is obviously named according to the does-what-it-says-on-the-tin format. Users refer to relationships as 'arrangements' or 'mutually beneficial relationships'. That's a euphemism for an arm's-length relationship between a wealthy, successful (and usually older) man and an attractive, entertaining and – most crucially – undemanding woman. Essentially the men pay for the luxury of a part-time, uncomplicated girlfriend. He gets a woman with youth and beauty who won't impinge on his life while she has access to a glamorous world of travel and elaborate restaurants, usually out of her reach, and most likely a designer wardrobe to boot. It's win-win.

As you will have gathered by now, I myself used so-called sugar daddy dating websites like this one. I used one with a less overt title – SugarDaddie.com – because I certainly wasn't looking for any sort of monetary 'arrangement' when I joined. I didn't even know such a culture existed. Aged 29, I was simply drawn by the promise of meeting an older, wiser, suited-and-booted type for cocktails and sophisticated conversation.

When I revealed that I had used sugar daddy dating sites in my book, *Sugar Daddy Diaries*, the charge from critics was that I must be a gold digger out to find a rich husband. In fact the opposite was true: I used these websites precisely because I didn't want a husband at all. The reason that I unwittingly found myself the recipient of gifts and luxury travel was because the men, I soon learned, considered it appropriate to provide some sort of compensation for what they couldn't offer emotionally. It seemed to me that such an explicit way of defining the boundaries of the relationship assuaged their guilt that they could not commit. Which, if you think about it, is far more honest than wooing a girl into bed, pretending to offer commitment and then disappearing into the sunset afterwards.

This is certainly the rationalism of 52-year-old Yushiro, Japanese-born, of Korean descent and raised in the US. Culturally he was somewhere between the three countries and didn't feel he belonged fully to any of them. His working life took him all over the world; he rarely stayed in one place for more than a week. He agreed to meet me so he could explain his reasons in full for seeking a 'mutually beneficial arrangement' instead of a conventional girlfriend.

Yushiro appeared to have a most gentle, easy-going temperament. His simple observations reminded me of the kind of tittle-tattle dear old ladies engage in. The temperature of his tea, the price of things in shop windows, the weather... sweet, innocent annotations, yet he led a far from cosseted life. One of the most powerful businessmen in Asia, his work led him to regularly meet Asian diplomats and VIPs but it meant he had no base. He had an ex-wife and children in America, who lived in the same town as his parents. Every few weeks he would return to the US and stay with his parents so that he could spend time with his children, but most of his life was spent in hotels.

Yushiro said he found it hard to nurture a circle of close friends, let alone a committed girlfriend. Until age 32, he'd only slept with one woman – his wife. Since his divorce he'd slept with dozens but he had only had one other love and that was Lucy, whom he paid to be his travelling companion in an arrangement that lasted five years.

'I met her in London at a party when she was a student,' Yushiro explained. 'At first I thought, "Wow, she's so tall and beautiful, she would never like me." Then our bodies brushed as she walked past and she seemed to like it, so I thought, "OK, I can talk to her." We got on – I couldn't believe she liked me. She said she liked to travel and I said I constantly travel for work and it sometimes gets lonely, so would she like to join me next time I travel? She was a student and said she couldn't afford to, so obviously I said I'd pay. There was no time to meet her first for a date to see if we got on – I'm only in a place for two or three days and then I'm off.

'We didn't discuss any sort of payment but when she arrived in Singapore I was working every day so I gave her some spending money so she could entertain herself in the daytime. I noticed that she didn't spend it and when I asked why, she was embarrassed and told me she needed the money just to live and didn't want to shop or go to expensive spas. I felt bad – how dreadful of me to assume how she wanted to spend her money. From then on I'd always give her a few thousand pounds whenever she came out to visit me. I called it "spending money" but I knew she'd spend it when she got home on the basic needs, like rent.

'I would say to her, "I have to spend four days in Delhi or

a week in San Francisco" and then I'd email her a ticket and we'd go. It was great! She told everyone I was her boss and she was my PA and had to travel around the world with me.' He paused and sighed before adding, 'I think I'm looking for my Lucy again.'

'What happened to her?'

'She emailed to say she had met someone serious. I was devastated but I understood. She's married to him now.'

'Does he know about you?'

'She will never tell him about me. I can understand that – I was flying her out to places all over the world and giving her pocket money to get her through college. He would not like to think of her like that.'

'Did you love her?'

Yushiro simply said Lucy was the only other proper relationship he had had, other than his wife. 'I could never think of the relationship as having a direction. She was only 25. With my life I can't have a serious girlfriend because I'm in this country and that country, and I have children in the States. When I got divorced it was only then that it dawned on me how much of a strain my travel was on my marriage. I had to live in Japan for a year and then South Korea – that's when my marriage broke down. After I got over my divorce I thought, "This is cool." I felt freedom.' He paused and then as an afterthought, alluded to Lucy again: 'She'll be 40 sometime around now, I think.'

Yushiro's language was simple and matter-of-fact. It was hard to detect whether he would like a more conventional loving relationship or if his mutually beneficial arrangements were enough for him. In a typically Japanese way he conceded that he couldn't have one and that was that; the question of want did not come into it.

Despite Yushiro's high profile and his five-star travel budget, his lifestyle was nomadic. He said English was now his first language over Japanese but his accent showed that his fluency was far from native speaker level. His parents spoke a pidgin Korean and Japanese but he had little in common with them and the rest of his family now. He grew up in Japan but hadn't been back for 20 years; he was of Korean descent but hostile immigration laws in Japan meant he could not have a Japanese passport, even though he spoke no Korean. To all intents and purposes he was nationality-less and base-less. For him a financial arrangement with a young and beautiful travel companion was the only romance he had the scope for.

* * *

Emily joined the site to look for a replacement benefactor after her previous arrangement came to an end. He was 25 years her senior and the relationship lasted a year, seeing each other a manageable three to four times a month. Divorced, he was unwilling to get into another serious relationship but enjoyed having a familiar and pretty face for one night out in the week and occasional weekends away in the South of France.

'I was living in Somerset with my mum when we met,' Emily began. The voluptuous brunette had once dreamed of being a model but now had her heart set on a career as a high-flying PA. 'I was visiting friends in London and I met him in a club. He told me he was separated from his wife and soon to be divorced. He took a real interest in me and I was flattered. He asked for my number and the following week he came all the way to Somerset to take me out. It was lovely to have everything paid for. We took things slowly at first and after two months he took me away to a fabulous country manor. I'd never been anywhere like it. I was aware of how much older he was so I wasn't thinking long-term, but he was so considerate and well mannered and took me to places no other boyfriend had.

'I remember once, when we were due to go away, I had an argument with my mum and she refused to take my dogs for the weekend so I was stuck with them. He was supposed to be picking me up that afternoon to take me away. I phoned him in tears and five minutes later, he called back to say he had found a hotel where we could bring the dogs with us! Then one day, around four months after we met, I confided in him the dire state of my finances. He didn't say anything but the next time we met, he produced a prepaid credit card so I could go out and get anything I needed. The relationship spiralled like that. Before I knew it, I was getting gifts left, right and centre. Then he offered to pay the rent for a flat so I could move out from living with my mum. He paid my bills and provided me with a car, plus the insurance.

'I didn't have any means of furnishing the flat so he bought kitchenware, rugs and bedding. Then he bought a laptop. He set me up so I could thrive independently. I have him to thank for everything I have now and for who I am. From what he provided I was able to go on to bigger and better things, build my confidence, apply for jobs.

'Once he started to fund my lifestyle, it became natural for me to ask for things. I wasn't in love but I grew to love him. I liked the fact that he liked me enough to treat me like this. I did start to think "maybe this could turn into something special" but I do question whether we ever would have got past three months if he hadn't provided so much for me.

'We split up after a holiday in New Orleans. I found out that he was still trying to make things work with his wife. Suddenly it felt like everything we had was invalid; I felt like he was having his cake and eating it. Although I benefited from him funding my lifestyle, I realised that this was his way of keeping me in a certain place. I felt like I'd been tagged along like a poodle. I realised that if you're paying someone then they can treat you how they want and you don't have the right to demand an explanation.

'When we split up I had to do everything by myself again – pay my own rent, my own car insurance, my own council tax. It was a real shock. But you know what?' She paused and her voice became shriller, as if she were about to reveal a hurtful truth: 'I now think that if I met someone who could provide for my lifestyle needs again, I'd be better off marrying them because then I'd know it would be more permanent.'

* * *

While I am sympathetic towards those who choose to have mutually beneficial relationships, it sounds like this wasn't really for Emily. The reason her benefactor or 'sugar daddy' was so grandiose with his generosity was precisely because he felt entitled to have a life outside of her. He was paying for freedom. Emily was clearly hurt that he was still contacting his ex-wife. My prognosis would be that she would have been better off seeking the rewards of her relationship in the currency of commitment rather than rent and furnishings.

I know what you're thinking. The parallels between these arrangements and prostitution are not lost on anyone, including members of the websites. This unfortunate analogy was the elephant in the online chat room. Men would say things like, 'There has to be mutual attraction otherwise this becomes "something else".' We all knew what the 'something else' referred to. But there is a transactional element to all relationships. One could probably map them on a sliding scale with hard and fast cash-for-sex on one end and the fanciful passions of romantic love on the other end. Neither promises much longevity but in the middle lie the tamer 'pragmatic relationships', where you can bet there will be some unspoken levelling of compromise and reward, such as commitment for companionship.

The royal mistress Nell Gwyn, who we met last chapter, was slandered as a 'whore' in front of crowds on many occasions but it didn't phase her. She once replied, 'I *am* a whore – find something else to fight about.' Nell clearly saw the bigger picture.

With mutually beneficial relationships or arrangements, sex is no greater part of the package than any romantic entanglement ultimately demands. In Japan there is an established practice known as *enjo-kosai*, which would translate as 'compensated dating'. A study by the Asian Women's Fund in 1998 found that more than 20 per cent of high-school girls engaged in *enjo-kosai* but 90 per cent said they would never involve themselves in sex for money. This shows that, for Japanese women, compensated dating is worlds apart from prostitution.

Enjo-kosai involves a young girl going out for dinner or karaoke with a much older man in exchange for material goods or money. Women's groups in Japan insist that it's the non-sexual activities that define *enjo-kosai*. Motives are as much to do with the fantasy surrounding the company of a young, perfumed, cherubic female than sex. I always used to get the feeling that the men I dated on sugar daddy sites wanted a glamorous woman as a sort of luxury status symbol, like an expensive car or a Montblanc pen – something he took pride and pleasure in looking after and treating with great care.

It's also telling that SeekingArrangment.com has ten times as many women than men, as it claims on its website. Compare that to 'no-strings' or adult dating websites, which have up to six times as many men than women. Both promote commitment-free relationships but only one has a materialistic incentive for women. I'm no rocket scientist but one-to-ten versus six-to-one? It's hard to argue that women don't need some sort of enticement for commitment-free sex.

Yet arrangements on sugar daddy sites like SeekingArragnment.com are not exploitative or dishonest. In fact I would argue they are quintessentially honest: each party defines what he or she wants. A 'sugar daddy' woos over a woman with material promises instead of emotional ones. It still fits the criteria for sexual selection theory in that both partners reap their gender-specific rewards. The man gets access to a sexual partner and the woman can be confident he can provide in some way. Admittedly this is no way to find a soul mate but that isn't what everybody wants from every relationship all of the time.

Of course there are other relationships based on 'arrangements' that are quite the opposite of the mutually beneficial relationship. Some arrangements are made not to allow both parties to keep their independence, but to make them completely accountable and dedicated to each other…

CHAPTER 13

Yes, Master

In early 2012 a print-on-demand book, by a little known virtual publisher, in a little known genre, shocked the literary world by becoming a bestseller. The prose was savaged by critics and the subject matter hardly mainstream, yet the first instalment of this lengthy trilogy went viral and by March 2012 it had become a *New York Times* bestselling eBook, set the record for the world's fastest selling paperback and started a craze for a new genre we now refer to as 'Mommy Porn'. What else could it be than E. L. James' *Fifty Shades of Grey*?

A great advert for self-publishing but an even better one for the mysterious world of dominant-submissive relationships, it generated column-metres. News stories abounded claiming BDSM (Bondage, Domination, Sadism and Masochism) clubs had seen a rise in first-timers and racy confessionals by outwardly looking normal couples revealing their secret kinky sex lives appeared. It seemed everyone wanted to have a go.

Well, definitely not me! I have to admit, I've always regarded anything to do with fetishes, skin-tight rubber, nipple clamping and whips and canes in dark dungeons as downright weird. The idea of mixing even a soupçon of pain with sex has never tickled my fancy. I can't help thinking that anyone who wants to inflict pain, be inflicted with pain, watch others be inflicted with pain, or who wants to walk on all fours wearing a dog collar has some seriously wonky screws. As for keeping one's loved one on a leash, how can such an exaggerated power imbalance bring the same rewards as a relationship based on parity and respect? Isn't dominance and submission simply a convenient mask for irreverent tyrants to brainwash vulnerable individuals and get off on it? You must admit, it certainly looks that way to outsiders. However, I now know it's more profound than that. Dominant-submissive relationships are all about conscious power manipulation, which requires a deep level of trust, intimacy, surrender and responsibility. For some people that's the most rewarding thing about the relationship.

Before I exemplify, let's get some of the lingo out of the way. Like the poly scene we visited in Chapter 10, the BDSM community has developed its own rich lexicon to reflect concepts that conventional couples wouldn't ever need to reference. In a dominant and submissive relationship, one party is known as the master or dominant while the other is the submissive or slave. It even has its own hieroglyphic: *D/s*, with the D for dominant always written in uppercase.

People outside of the BDSM community are known as 'vanilla'. Those who enjoy dabbling in both submissive and dominant role-play are called 'switches'. 'Play' is the term used for the physical or erotic acts between BDSM couples. Note: I didn't say sexual. Whether BDSM is sexual is a pedantic debate within the community. Play *can* include sex but it might just be a good beating. Some people on the BDSM scene refuse to call it a sexual practice because they view the two as totally different experiences. Others point out that the sexualised imagery associated with BDSM – the exposure of flesh, the focus on genitalia and the frequency with which play evokes sexual arousal indicates that, of course, it overlaps with erotic fantasies.

As one BDSM enthusiast said, 'It is often the sexual fantasies that sub-dom role-playing evokes, rather than physical stimulation.' She then exemplified with a story of a friend who allows a man to visit her home once a week and clean it from top to bottom, naked. She doesn't pay him. But it goes further than that. *He* leaves *her* a present, as a symbol of his submission. 'What he does when he goes home who knows, but certainly there's nothing sexual when he's at her house,' she surmised.

Some couples have an otherwise normal romantic dynamic but only take on the D/s dynamic during play. Others, like same-sex couple Lesley and Cate, conduct their entire relationship in dominant-submissive role-play – a 24-7 relationship.

Lesley, 35, works as an administrator at a small local company near Leicester and has the luxury of working from home three days a week. Cate, 32, is a property solicitor and works long hours at a local law firm, also in Leicester, where they both live. They have been together for five years and legal civil partners for three.

Aside from Cate's solid silver neck-collar, the pair gave nothing away to suggest their connection to the BDSM scene. Both had short dark hair and were of average height, dressed casually in jeans and black tops. I spoke to each of them separately so I could garner an unsolicited account of their interaction. 'Basically I am in charge,' explained Lesley. 'I can say, "Don't do that" and she can't. She has the right to say no whenever she wants and I'd never ask her to do things she isn't comfortable with.' Lesley spoke with a mild West Country accent. Calm and controlled, her voice carried little expression.

She was introduced to the BDSM scene by an ex girlfriend, who took her to one of the UK's best-known fetish clubs called Club AntiChrist in London. Having grown up in a small village in the country it had never occurred to her to visit a fetish club but she found herself enjoying it and so they introduced dominant-submissive role-play during sex. She said she naturally fell into the submissive role. Now, however, she's the one in the driving seat.

She met Cate in her local pub four years ago when Cate was visiting university friends. They exchanged emails but didn't meet until six months later and soon settled into a relationship. Cate initially knew nothing of Lesley's BDSM past but then the secret was thrown into the open.

'One evening when Cate and I had only been going out a few weeks, we went to a birthday meal. We were late and when we arrived, one of my friends joked to Cate, "Did she have you tied up and was she spanking you again?" They just presumed Cate was into the same things as me! Cate looked a little shocked but just laughed. But on the way home, she pulled me up on it and so I told her about that side of me.'

'I was surprised,' said Cate later, when I asked for her version. 'But I didn't think it was an issue. I'd read about

BDSM and although I'd never actually sought it, I did have an interest on some level.'

The next time Lesley went to a fetish club she invited Cate, who accepted with nervous excitement: 'There were eight or nine rooms with various pieces of kit. There were medical rooms with hospital beds for medical play, posts for people to be chained to; there were sterile needles for temporary piercings. I found it exciting rather than shocking,' Cate reflected. 'People engaged in heavy or light play as they wished. Some people want to be hit until they are screaming on the floor, others want to be hit just until it starts to hurt.' Despite the graphic nature, Cate decided she liked it and so they made fetish clubs a regular part of their social life. Over time, their sex life increasingly featured BDSM. They moved in together three months after Cate's first BDSM introduction and Lesley said she found herself unwittingly giving Cate orders outside of the bedroom as well as inside. Cate seemed to take delight in complying.

'It started with me giving her foods that she didn't like and making her eat [them] five times a week,' Lesley recalled. 'She grew up in a household which never tried anything new, so she'd written off a whole load of food. She didn't even eat pasta until she was 21! One evening she turned her nose up at olives. I made her eat a couple and we laughed about it and I said, sort of jokingly, "You have to eat olives three times a day for two weeks." We found ourselves sticking with it, and it was fun enforcing it.

'Then I told her that she could only drink three times a week. When we met, she drank every night and that's not healthy. She wasn't happy about it – she asked for more nights than three. I said no. There are some weeks when she'll request more nights. I'll ask her why, and she'll have to present her reasons. It might be that she's meeting friends for dinner or has a work function. I'll assess and then say yes or no.

'Then I brought in things like orgasm control. I'd say, "No masturbating this week", and so she could only orgasm with me. The little rules crept in at first. Only when I realised that Cate liked it, did I sit her down and say, "What do you think about making this a 24-7 lifestyle?" I told her very clearly that it might mean there would be things she couldn't do anymore. Would she be happy with that? And she was. We revisit the rules often. If I notice she's tired and snappy, I'll say, "Are you sure you want to be in this sort of relationship, or do you just want to be my wife?" The important thing with a sub-dom connection is communication.'

In a 24-7 relationship, the submissive partner or 'slave' often wears an irremovable collar to symbolise dedication to their master. They even have collaring ceremonies. Lesley and Cate had theirs on the same day as their wedding. When the civil ceremony at the registry office was over, they went to their favourite fetish club, where Cate was confirmed as the submissive property of her wife Lesley. The owner of the club conducted the 'service' in front of around 20 of their friends, most of them alien to the BDSM scene. Cate was on her knees throughout. Once she gave her affirmation that she would be the submissive property of Lesley, she was ceremoniously fitted with a silver necklace sealed at the back with a small screw, only ever to be removed with a special tool.

The collar soon got them into trouble on their honeymoon to Turkey. 'The airport security guard asked her to remove it and she refused. He said "Why?" and Cate said, "Because it doesn't come off,"' Lesley giggled.

'It isn't what you might imagine – that the submissive does all the cleaning and I put my feet up,' she resumed. 'We are egalitarian when it comes to domesticity. She works more hours so I do more housework. We both give to the relationship as much as each other. Emotionally I'm there for her all the time. Most of my rules are things that I think Cate will benefit from. If she comes home after a long day and looks tired, I'll say go and put jeans on because she looks like she needs to. Or I'll say, "Go to bed", and then she can't do anything else. If guests are with us, I'll tell her to make tea but many couples ask the other one to do that anyway. I wouldn't ask her to do things that she wouldn't do off her own back.

'I make her exercise too. It was her own idea to sign up to a gym but I make sure she goes. She talks through her training programme with me and we draw something up suited to her. I don't dictate when she goes, but if we're going out I might object or I'll call her and tell her to stop what she's doing and come home, and she will.'

Already I could feel myself recoil. If a boyfriend (or girlfriend, if I were that way inclined) made me cut a gym session short, I would probably take a dumbbell home and throw it at them.

'We only have two arbitrary rules: first, she has to stand up when I come into the room. It's to symbolise that this is a power-dynamic relationship. Second, she can't sit unless I tell her to; that's absolute. If people come to visit they wouldn't notice because I do it so subtly – with a nod or a pat of the chair. The only time I relax that rule is when we're in public. On a bus, for instance, it's just awkward if Cate is standing in someone's way waiting for me to tell her to sit down. It inconveniences other people, and that's not why we have this relationship: for us, it's the fact that we know we have this power dynamic, which is part of who we are and how we are with each other.'

Lesley hadn't always called the shots in relationships. Before she met Cate her D/s activities had been limited to the bedroom and she had played both the sub and the dom. Which begs the question, how did she adapt to becoming such a bossy boots with the person she loves without letting guilt gnaw away?

'It's a question I look into often,' she answered. 'It isn't something I tried to create in previous relationships and I've never been an over-assertive person. I've had lots of vanilla relationships and I never felt anything was missing. I always say to Cate, "If you're unhappy, I need to know." I love her more than anything else in the world. There are times when she doesn't like what I tell her to do. The first time I told her to eat a full chicken breast, it took an hour and she cried through the whole thing. She wanted my approval, yes, but also somewhere in her brain she knows that being a fussy eater is restrictive and she wants to change that. When you really don't want to do something and you make yourself do it, you feel good because you know that you've endured something.'

On that note, if the attraction of being bossed around is the sense of accomplishment in doing something you can't motivate yourself to do, maybe how much we enjoy a relationship is down to how we motivate ourselves. Personally I have no problem making myself do things I don't want to do. In fact, the majority of my life is spent in this way! Every morning I force myself to jog to the gym. Sometimes it's snowing and it's dark. Once there, there are more pain barriers. Come to think about it, I spend the first two hours of every day screaming to myself, 'Just 40 seconds more!' Then there's more pain barriers when I sit at my desk to work. Sometimes the whole day is a big battle against ennui – cleaning the loo and eating my greens because these are things we have to do. Thankfully I don't need a dominant partner to make me do them.

It did make me wonder whether there's another sliding scale at play here. On one end of it there are those who gladly submit themselves to the control of a partner because they can't take responsibility for themselves. Then on the other end there are the headstrong contented singletons like me, who'd probably want to punch someone's lights out if they tried to tell us what to do. In the middle are your everyday couples, who find being in a relationship comforting because it provides them with just the nudge they need to navigate life as best they can.

Cate confirmed she enjoyed being assuaged of self-responsibility – 'When Lesley started banning things, I knew it was good for me so I didn't mind.' She spoke with a Newcastle accent, her tone unsentimental at first. She warmed up gradually, then her voice relaxed and gave way to an occasional shy giggle. 'We were visiting London one weekend and Lesley bought me a leather collar to show me I was hers. She said she wanted me to wear it when we were together. I was really proud to have it and I wore it all the time – I hadn't been in a proper relationship before, I'd just dated people and had one-night stands. The fact that she bought me a collar indicated we were getting on a more permanent footing. It was like being given a key to the house. I was delighted. When Lesley noticed I didn't take it off, she said, "Oh, do you want the whole lifestyle thing?' That's when we started to talk about going 24-7. I did have concerns but mainly about who would know. I'm a private person and there's a view that BDSM people are perverts, so I wanted control over that. We talked through all sorts of things – that's why my collar is silver, not leather, because it can pass as a nice necklace.'

'Didn't you worry about losing your autonomy and choice?' I asked.

'No, because I knew that if I wasn't happy, Lesley would act on that. I like having things decided for me – it makes life easier. At work I have lots of authority and control, and I like not having that when I come home. The cliché is that submissives allow themselves to be treated that way because they are playing out past scenes of abuse but I don't think that's the case. I had an idyllic childhood with a stable, loving home. The only issue I ever had was coming out as gay, but that wasn't a massive deal.

'I know Lesley would never do anything that would put me in danger or overstep what I'm comfortable with. By the time we entered into 24-7 she knew enough about me to know how far to push me. Because we've discussed my boundaries I know some things just aren't on the table. One thing I said I wouldn't do is humiliation – I had a bad time at school and it would trigger memories. And I don't want permanent marks on my skin either. The difference between BDSM and abuse is consent, so if she ever crossed the line of what I'd consented to, I would just leave.'

Both managed to have a giggle about their dynamic. Some of the things Lesley tells Cate to do are apparently 'for her own amusement'. When asked to elaborate, Lesley said she sometimes makes Cate strike up a conversation with strangers. Her task is to find out as much as she can about them. Lesley finds it funny to watch and Cate believes it's 'good for her' because it's helped her to overcome shyness.

'I turned her into a birthday card once,' giggled Lesley. 'I tied her naked and blindfolded to a pole in a club and gave everyone a marker pen so they could sign her.' Another time Lesley made Cate pretend to be a hamster and gave her a giant water bottle filled with beer, which she had to drink over a night out.

By now you are probably thinking the same as me: that sounds dangerously close to humiliation, one of the lines that Cate did not wish to cross. But she sees everything Lesley does as being for her own sake: 'I've been healthier since being with Lesley. She'll point out things that make me tired and grumpy that I don't see myself and she's good at seeing when I'm stressed.' So what would happen if Cate broke the rules, or if she grew sick of being told what to do and snapped back? 'I wouldn't,' she replied without hesitation. 'Because dominance and submission are about trust and if either breaks that, it's hard to get it back. If I want to do something that I'm not meant to, I have a rational conversation with Lesley. Sometimes she lets me and sometimes she doesn't. But sneaking off and doing it would be a breach of trust – Lesley would be really upset.

'When we first started with 24-7 she told me to go to bed because I looked tired. I went upstairs but she heard me turn the computer on and wow, she was upset! It was a wake-up call to me about how serious she is about these roles. It upset me to see how bad I made her feel – I wouldn't do that again.'

Cate was relieved to hand her self-responsibilities to someone else. She trusted her partner's decisions more than her own but as she points out, this is not dissimilar to the mechanisms of many modern marriages: 'I listen to my colleagues talk about their husbands and wives and it's just the same,' she said, releasing one of her nervous giggles. 'They have things that are expected of them. With my boss, it's so obvious that his wife is in charge. He's not allowed to turn his mobile off. If he doesn't answer she'll ring his work phone and if he doesn't answer that, she'll ring other people around the office to see where he is. It's not even for important stuff! Usually it's something like, did he remember to hand in the consent form for the school trip? My boss sometimes says to me, "I'm in trouble again, Cate, because I had to take work home last night." But he's smiling when he says it – he seems to quite enjoy it. BDSM just takes these power dynamics and exaggerates them.'

* * *

But exaggeration can go too far. Robert, a 31-year-old schoolteacher, is apprehensive about 24-7 D/s relationships after being in one for five years with his girlfriend, whom he met at 18. They had already been together for five years before they adopted the D/s lifestyle and stayed that way for a further five years. Robert played the submissive and his girlfriend, it seems, played a sexually insatiable dominatrix.

'I'm more dominant than submissive by character but I also really enjoyed being submissive in my last relationship. In a way they are the same in terms of appeal – it's the same fantasy viewed from different angles,' Robert said. He was handsome with dark Mediterranean looks, thick black hair and a toned physique.

'We played with something called domestic servitude. If I didn't perform certain daily chores, there would be complete hell to pay. I would be put into a torture device, where my legs were spread and I had small electric tweezers applied to my testicles. Or I would be put on a 'Queening Stool', which restricts movement so you have to orally pleasure the dominant on top.' He spoke confidently and fluently, brushing aside any embarrassment to be informative.

'We also did a lot of denial games so for instance, I wasn't allowed to orgasm. That meant I was totally reliant on her to do it for me. I wore a discrete chastity belt every day, even at work. Giving her complete control of my sexual needs would send me into a frenzied horn – I'd have an astonishing orgasm, hypnotic almost.

'I enjoyed it while it lasted but we fell out of love. It took us a while to realise that if you strip away that dynamic, there wasn't much left. I wouldn't want that extreme again. If we had paused for thought, we probably wouldn't have prolonged it for as long as we did. When we got together, we didn't have intentions to enter BDSM or do anything kinky; It started as an experiment. I always think you get the best of a situation when you don't go too far. It's like drugs – you can have a bit and it's enjoyable in moderation but if you do it too much, there are consequences.

'You become in danger of losing the magic you had with that person. With BDSM you get to see dark things from the dark corners of your partner's mind. They see yours too, which are very often taboo things. It can alter your perception. You start to think, "I'm not sure about this person any more because I know that they are this way inclined." It changes the dynamic between you permanently; it creeps up. My girlfriend looked up to me in the beginning. I helped her get into college, get her first job; I gave her confidence and brought about good things in her life. By the end, I'd spent so long playing the submissive that she didn't look up to me as she once did.'

That was only three years ago and Robert was now engaged to a 21-year-old aspiring model called Stacy. They too gravitated towards dominant-submissive role playing, but after his last experience, Robert was adamant that he would keep it in the bedroom this time and not let it overspill into other areas of the relationship.

'She knew about my past and I think she was intrigued. She'd never tried BDSM but when she read *Fifty Shades of Grey*, she told me she'd like to try some things. It just worked for us – we were looking for something more exciting in the bedroom and it took off.

'It started with things like teasing and denial. We play certain games leading up to sex. Like, we'll have foreplay but she's not allowed to come. She then becomes really eager to please. I'll ask her to perform acts on herself and dance for me and then tell her to stop when she nearly reaches climax. I get lots of enjoyment from watching her – she's very beautiful and if I'm denying her an orgasm that really gets her going and frustrated.

'We started a bit of pain play but not in the extreme sense – we don't do flogging or nipple clamps. I suppose we do lots of things that are considered taboo: anal sex and bondage. Her tolerance to the pain increases the more we do but even so, I don't want to spoil it.'

Over time, though, Robert conceded, bedroom play did creep into their domestic lives and he constantly monitors things so their dynamic doesn't start to affect their feelings for each other, as it did with his previous relationship. 'We started playing around a bit with servitude and domestic discipline so she has to do things around the house, sometimes dressed in sexy outfits. I'd never take it outside of the home – I have such high regard for her, I would never embarrass her in public – but I might do very subtle things like I'll tell her she has to present herself immaculately and call me "Sir" when we're out for dinner. It's so discrete no one else would know. With my past relationship we continually pushed each other until we were doing things way out of our comfort zones in public and I look back and feel bad about that.'

Having played dominant and submissive, Robert is convinced that counterintuitively, it's the submissive who gets the best deal: 'During play, I have to keep things interesting but at the same time monitor her safety. Her welfare lies in my hands. I have to really concentrate. I'm judging her boundaries and thinking of the creative aspect at the same time. It is a joy, but it's also a stress. She's my angel – I'd die if anything happened to her. I have to find that zone where it feels unsafe for her because that's what she wants but really is quite safe. I do a lot of prep for our games and I test things on myself first. If I use candle wax, a few hours before I'll drip it onto the table from different heights and test the heat with my elbow. Everything I do is designed with her stimulation in mind.

'The idea that the dominant calls the shots isn't entirely true. You actually find that submissives are the ones that dictate how the play goes because they set the limits and everything is being done according to their preferences. Because I love her so much, I don't want to take advantage so when we're out of sub-dom mode I find myself making it up to her ten-fold. I'll pay her lots of attention, bring her drinks, rub her feet... There'll be lots of cuddles and caring talk.'

* * *

There's certainly no danger of becoming bored on the BDSM scene. A quick skim of any forum or networking group gives a glimpse of the popular themes for 'play'. Domestic servitude, as Robert educated us, is one of the tamer ones. Sometimes the tasks required of the slave are as bland as dusting or fixing refreshments. Then there's 'human furniture', when the submissive takes on the duties and shape of a piece of furniture for a length of time decided by their master. If they get off lightly, they may get to be a kneeling footstool but they could equally end up becoming a coffee table withstanding mugs of hot tea on the flat of their back while their master watches TV. Or perhaps a hanging light fitting or a sliding wardrobe door. The opportunities are endless.

It gets murkier, the deeper you delve. Erotic humiliation, for instance, is where one partner is sexually demeaned in front of a crowd. Dodgier sounding still is 'sexual slavery', where the dominant partner has the prior-agreed consent of the submissive to request whatever sexual acts they like for however long they want. Teetering on the edge of what could be illegal or insane is something called 'edge play', a term for anything which pushes the boundaries of safe, sane and consensual (SSC). Edge play includes erotic asphyxiation, fire, knife and gun play. Some even derive a thrill from the risk of spreading disease by cutting (sometimes known as blood play) or bareback sex with an infected partner. Wow!

As I spoke to more and more people on the BDSM scene, I started to see that submissive and dominant role playing appears to be a tool to form a deep connection. It's not the act of submitting or dominating per se, which gives pleasure, it's the raw emotion that it drags with it. Dominants expose their primal fantasies and submissives peel away tough exteriors to expose their weaknesses and fears.

Hannah and her fiancé Craig, both 30, exemplified this best. They met five years ago through a local BDSM networking group in the Northwest. Hannah is an office administrator and Craig works in retail. They're an average-looking couple. Hannah is short and heavily built, with long strawberry blonde hair tied back loosely. Craig towers above her, bald with glasses and tattooed arms. When I met them they were planning their wedding and hoped to start a family soon after. They were both confident that their BDSM lifestyle would 'always be a part of them' even after they have children.

They were sitting side by side on the sofa, looking relaxed, Craig's arm outstretched on the top of the cushions and his fingers resting on Hannah's shoulders. 'When you enter into submission, you give yourself up to someone else,' he explained. 'For a window of time, your reactions are no longer a response to yourself. Someone has to look after you. It's a retrograde move to a childlike state – you're being cared for and you don't have to take responsibility for your needs. Some people say they like feeling that whatever they are doing is to please someone else. It's the closest you'll ever get to selflessness. Being submissive is not the same with one person as another, even if the mechanics of what is happening to them look the same.'

Hannah nodded in agreement. 'It's called sub space,' she said cheerfully. 'It's a psychological space you go to when you've gone past the pain barrier and are being deeply submissive. Some people may reach it through meditation or yoga. The further down you go, the more compliant you will get and that's when the Dom has to be confident that they know what the sub really wants because if they are that far under, what they say they want may not really be what they want. That's why it's essential to talk beforehand. I personally wouldn't be confident taking someone down that deep who I didn't know extremely well.'

Hannah described sub space as 'a sort of intoxicated state, minus the drugs'. She made constant reference to 'going under', 'going down deep' and someone who 'had never gone that far into sub space before', as if it were a physical place in the subconscious mind. I had heard others talk similarly. Lesley had described an 'endorphin high, like the floaty feeling when you've pushed yourself through exercise and gone past the pain barrier'.

'But can you really enjoy pain?' I very rationally asked.

'I can find the sensation of pain pleasurable in the right circumstances,' answered Craig. 'Not if I drop a book on my foot but if I'm in the middle of a scene and what is happening is painful, I can enjoy that. I enjoy getting past the pain barrier – it's the sense of relief that is enjoyable.' Then he added: 'Our play isn't necessarily about pain: it's the reaction that's the key. I'll happily tickle Hannah rather than hit her because it's her response that I look for. I enjoy the softer side of things – what people refer to as "sense playing" – because I can get lost in it. If you are creating pain, you have to concentrate much harder because you are focusing on not causing real damage.' He turned to Hannah and smiled, inviting her to comment.

'If I'm being beaten or something like that, once you've gone through your pain control, you reach the eye of the storm, where it doesn't hurt any more and then it is the most relaxing, cathartic feeling you can find. It's amazing, actually.

Pain is a simple thing to control – it's a matter of breathing and telling your head not to panic.' Hannah's eyes lit up as she talked. She clearly had more to share.

'My first few years in BDSM were when I played the hardest. I had wanted to try it for a long time so I revelled in it and many times I ended up with injuries for longer than I expected. Once, I went to work after barely any sleep and I had scratches and bruises all over me, even the bits outside of my clothes – I found it exhilarating. Another time I had bruises on my butt cheeks for three weeks after I'd been beaten very hard while wearing a tight skirt. I found it highly amusing.' She turned to Craig, her eyes still wide, and smiled mischievously. He rolled his eyes affectionately and reminded me that all these activities were 'way before they met'. 'There was no lasting damage and I like having marks anyway,' she concluded

If being flogged in sub space is really so magical, maybe we should be asking what the dominant gets out of it. So, is there a dom-space? 'That's also different for different people,' answered Craig. 'When I'm dominating, I like that I am responsible for someone, that I'm caring for them and giving them an experience that they enjoy. But it can also be about exploring – helping someone find limits they didn't know they had. Helping them to get to know about themselves as a person. There is so much more to it than what people get through just sex.'

The pair first tried to keep their D/s play in the bedroom but, according to Hannah, it's easier said than done: 'In theory our BDSM activities are purely for our sex life but in reality, you can't help it creeping into other areas of your relationship. It becomes part of your mindset, your language, how you see the world and interact with people.'

Both had got into BDSM in their twenties. Craig went through 'a Gothic stage' and found the BDSM scene was the best way he could experiment sexually with the types of women he was drawn to. For Hannah it was far simpler: 'It was the idea of kinky sex,' she said frankly. 'When I read fiction or watched films I always found the scenes with someone in pain or bound quite attractive, even if they weren't meant to be. I just knew – that side of me has always been there.'

They regularly attend fetish clubs and parties, play in people's homes and go to workshops. Play is sexual with each other but chaste with others. Hannah goes to rope-play classes with friends once a week, which she finds 'hugely relaxing' – 'I enjoy the task of tying someone up – it clears my head. There's a real skill to rope play and to whipping someone. I like the challenge of trying to whip someone in the way I want, to create damage in the way I want to, or they want.'

'What sort of damage?' I wanted to know.

'Red marks in certain places; shapes and patterns even. Or the way that the whip falls and the noises it makes. Getting the reaction you expected – there is a sense of achievement in it. Technique is important, you can't just wade in if you don't know what you're doing. If it's hitting or whipping then you should stick to backs of thighs and bottoms and avoid the kidney area or anywhere near the windpipe. If you are playing with canes and you don't mind marks, then the bottoms of feet, hands or the tops of arms are best – you have to be considerate that they need to get up and go to work the next day.

'I couldn't do vanilla sex now,' she concluded. 'It's in my instincts to dominate or allow someone to dominate me. I wouldn't know how *not* to bite or scratch. It would be like taking all of someone's sexual moves that they've been doing for years and years, and asking them not to do them.'

* * *

BDSM has a beatnik image but power play is a popular topic with which to capture the public imagination, even if we don't call it that. The 2013 film *Behind the Candelabra* starring Matt Damon and Michael Douglas was based on the true story of a controlling relationship between the pianist Liberace and his much younger lover, Scott Thorson. Liberace holds all the power, both in the bedroom and out of it. Eventually his young amour becomes so reliant on the affections and financial rewards of his elder, controlling master that he cannot leave even if he wants to.

In Nine and a Half Weeks, Mickey Rourke and Kim Basinger play a new couple with a volatile sex life. What started out as fun becomes control and then abuse; eventually it leads to the heroine's emotional breakdown.

But in reality does power play always lead to such a negative outcome? The BDSM community are quick to define the difference between play and personal abuse with two words: consent and intent. Their distinction is black and white, which is perhaps why every single person I spoke to within the BDSM community hated *Fifty Shades of Grey*, the consensus being that it was 'abusive'. Hannah was particularly disgusted by it: 'Christian Grey took a naive woman who had never had sex. He pushed her way beyond what she was willing to do. He didn't let her talk, which is very important in a master-slave relationship. In the third book there is a scene where he gets cross with her because she safe-worded. That wouldn't happen in this community – you can't give someone a safety net and then say they're a bad person for using it.'

There has been much research into the psychology of the dominant-submissive mindset but no evidence to suggest anyone with a preference for it has psychological problems. Yet they are still viewed with suspicion and often considered deviant or even ridiculed. Headlines such as 'X Caught Taking Part in Sick Sex Game', or 'Sex Game Gone Wrong' highlight the media's sensationalised view of this unconventional relationship model. There was little sympathy for ex-motorsport head Max Mosley when caught on video in 2011 acting out a Nazi scene with five prostitutes. The press revelled in 'Nazi Orgy' headlines, even though there was nothing to say anything sexual took place.

In the past, psychiatrists regarded activities relating to sadomasochism, bondage or dominance and submission as an illness. Hardly surprising if you consider that much tamer things, including homosexuality and female disobedience have also been classified as officially loony. It was only in 1994, with the release of the fourth version of the DSM (in case you have forgotten that ugly acronym, the DSM is the mental health diagnostic manual of internationally recognised disorders), when the psychiatric profession became more forgiving. The new DSM IV stated that BDSM was only a disorder if any of the associated behaviour caused distress, similarly to how asexuality is viewed. Like asexuality, campaigners have tried to have it removed altogether. They say that 'stress' might be caused from the stigma of their sexual preferences rather than the preferences themselves.

Denmark, Sweden, Norway and Finland are the only

European countries to have removed all association with BDSM and psychiatric disorders. But social acceptance is widening. Many relationship therapists and counsellors now make a point of advertising if they are 'BDSM aware'. Even the charity Relate advertises that some of its counsellors are 'kink friendly'.

Dr Charley Ferrer, a clinical sexologist, psychotherapist and herself a BDSM practitioner, has spent 15 years participating in and researching the BDSM lifestyle. She now works with medical professionals in America and Latin America to educate them on the kink lifestyle.

'I distinguish between a sadist in a dominance and submission role and a sadist, who is a pathological criminal based on their intent,' she explained. 'The pathology lies in the motivation behind the actions. For those who practise dominance and submissions in a role-play environment the intent is not to injure their partner but to experience intense intimacy and a more profound, spiritual, physical and erotic connection.

'If someone is maliciously trying to injure their partner or inciting psychological torment because they are angry or they have an issue with men or women, or because it gets them off, that's when there is a need for intervention because they could be acting as a criminal sadist.'

Dr Ferrer believes that there is a level of interest in BDSM for everyone. In her book *BDSM: The Naked Truth* she developed what she calls the 'Kinky Scale', named after the better-known 'Kinsey Scale', which the late Alfred Kinsey used to rate a person's 'degree of hetero and homo sexuality' from 0–6. 'In the Kinky Scale, level zero is for individuals who are strictly vanilla and who have no interest in dominance and submission, no desire and no fantasies,' she explained. 'Like Alfred Kinsey's scale, Dr Ferrer predicts that most people fit into the next one, Level One: you might have had a fantasy about it, it looks a little fun but no way will you interact with it. Then at Level Two, people are a little interested. They may try a bit of bondage or blindfolding – they taste the flavour of it but they don't identify as being part of BDSM. At Level Three, people are participating in it regularly and enjoying it. They probably have a partner or friend who practises it too. Level Four are those who actually embrace master-slave relationships. They feel this sort of relationship is right for them and that's how they want to conduct their relationships. Level Five individuals are edge players – they push things as far as they can go. Then there's Level Six, which is when people are pathological criminal sadists. These are people who should never be in the lifestyle to begin with and they sometimes enter the lifestyle to hide their abusive nature.'

As well as the danger of being pathologised, BDSM partakers have also been criminalised. One of the most famous cases was Operation Spanner in 1987. Manchester City police obtained a video of a large group taking part in BDSM. Convinced that the tied and gagged people in the video were being tortured before being killed, they launched a huge operation, raiding properties and making multiple arrests. The alleged victims assured police that they were willing participants, but nevertheless the police and the Crown Prosecution Service pressed charges and 16 people were convicted of all sorts of offences, including assault and actual bodily harm.

To me, control and domination are the things I find most threatening about a full-time committed relationship. For the contented singletons we met in Chapter One, wanting to maintain control is central to why they stay single. Episodes of what I call 'couple-control' are what I find to be the most ugly by-product of modern relationships and most at odds with our increasingly autonomous society. I consider control and forced unity to be the ticking time bomb of modern relationships yet D/s couples seize on control and play with it. It is the basis of their relationships. For them the exaggerated power dynamic heightens intimacy and locks them together. Their closeness rests on how they surrender themselves and how they trust each other to respect barriers.

Looking into BDSM was like placing a magnifying glass on the paradox of relationships: the more closeness you want to achieve, the more autonomy and self-identity must be surrendered.

CHAPTER 14

Mail-order Marriages

There is a saying in French, *Ceci n'empêche pas cela*, which means that just because you believe one thing, it doesn't necessarily mean you disagree with the opposite. So just because I don't search desperately and endlessly for a life-long partner to complete me, it doesn't mean that I wouldn't dismiss a man who came along who fascinated me, inspired me and whose company I adored. There is no vacancy for a boyfriend but that doesn't mean I wouldn't create a role if someone had a lot to offer.

Some people work in reverse, however. They start with a vacancy and find the person to fit it. For them companionship is more important than the companion. So important is it to them that they are willing to pay and travel thousands of miles to find a type they can easily mould. I met 25 men who were doing just that on a package tour to the Ukrainian town of Odessa.

Some call Odessa 'Rio for Russians' because there are plenty of women and plenty of places to party – if you have money. Others call it the 'Pearl of the Black Sea' because away from the shanty buildings on the outskirts, there is a quaint town centre with cobbled streets and historic buildings. In summer, al fresco bars come to life whereas in winter, the Black Sea becomes a solid block of white ice with the shapes of the waves intact, providing perfect ice bumps for children's sledges.

Mostly foreigners and expats are found in the bars and cafes, though. Ukraine – formerly part of the USSR – has been on the brink of bankruptcy for half a decade. Average salaries were £230 a month in 2011 according to the State Statistics Committee of Ukraine and even the highest earning doctor takes home no more than around £500 monthly. There is little disposable income for sipping espressos on cobbled streets. Odessa's main industry is tourism: more specifically, *marriage* tourism.

On my visit in the month of February, the mercury sunk to below -22. At that temperature the moisture inside your nostrils starts to freeze. Imagine then what happens to the lip gloss plastered on the 100 beautiful, skinny, educated young ladies gathering outside the Palladium nightclub at one in the afternoon in sheer tights, five-inch heels and just a faux fur over their cocktail dresses. Any blemishes from the biting cold were perfectly primed with thick lashings of foundation.

I watched the girls queue from the warmth of a coach, along with a group of men from Britain, Europe and America. They too had made an effort – handkerchiefs in top pockets, ironed shirts, expensive cufflinks, best aftershave. They didn't leer, they didn't whistle, they didn't shout 'phwoar!' – these men were serious. After all, they'd paid nearly £3,000 to be there and were set on finding a wife.

I'd been invited to join the trip by AnastasiaDate.com to

write a piece for a Sunday newspaper. The website connects men in affluent countries with women in former Soviet states and Latin America. Four times a year it organises what it calls 'romance tours' so members can meet the girls in person. For that price they get flights, accommodation and a 'concierge' to set up dates on their behalf. They are guaranteed at least one date a day, if they want it. But they may not need it because the package also includes organised trips to 'socials', which is where our bus had just delivered us.

Everyone in the town of Odessa knows what a social is. There is one nearly every Sunday and any female over 18 will have attended one. A social, you see, is some girls' only hope of ever getting out of this corrupt, chauvinistic, freezing country.

The men piled off and were ushered straight into the Palladium nightclub, bypassing the sea of women waiting patiently but eagerly for security to let them in. Twenty-five men, 100 women: that takes the sex ratio to four girls to every man. You may ask why such a smorgasbord of beautiful women would make themselves available for such a limited number of comparatively clapped-out older guys. And that would be a very good question. There are a number of reasons and theories behind this. First, there is a gender imbalance in Ukraine. Statistics vary across different ages but the overall male/female ratio in 2012 was 0.85, which means that for every male there are 1.17 females. Some historians put this down to the migration of young men from small towns into bigger cities or into mainland Russia, where they can earn more. Others put it down to the high number of men enlisted into military service. Another theory is that a high level of alcohol causes a chromosome imbalance in sperm, leading to the birth of more women. A less scientific sounding theory still is that in tough environments with high death rates, nature produces more women.

Next comes Ukraine's archaic cultural attitudes. Being single and a female past 25 is likened to unwanted Christmas cake (no one wants it after the 25th). Also, there are not many jobs for women beyond the traditionally female and lowly paid professions such as beauticians, carers or cleaners. Few Ukrainian women therefore can financially support themselves. This makes an older foreign husband, who is reasonably presentable, a viable marriage option.

Whatever the reason for the high number of available females, for men like Richard, a chatty, average-looking 52-year-old divorced entrepreneur from Seattle, it is worth flying 6,000 miles for: 'You walk into that room and suddenly all your insecurities disappear and you can join the buffet – a buffet of caviar. It's like picking your custom-made dream girl. You can take all the feminine traits you most like and look for one who has them all,' he said on the coach, his eyes sparkling.

Inside the vast Palladium nightclub, 'Brown Girl in the Ring' was playing as a compère invited both sexes onto the stage to play party games such as 'Pass the Balloon Between Your Legs' and something else involving a blindfold, which did not look like Pin the Tail on the Donkey. But while the backdrop might be tawdry, the men's intentions were not. For Matt, coming abroad to find a wife was a carefully considered assessment of odds. At 35, he had lived on the family ranch in Texas all his life. 'There aren't many women in ranch country,' he drawled. 'They've either moved to the cities or they are already married. All the ones that are left are of questionable morals.' He then proceeded to tell me story after story of adulterous women he'd found in beds, cars and outbuildings with other men.

Then there was Jeremy, a 47-year-old attorney from Mountain View in Silicon Valley. Known for its IT industry, the region attracts mainly male workers and so has the inverse gender imbalance as Ukraine – there is a shortage of women. Jeremy was by far the best-looking man on the romance tour. Glamorous twenty-somethings hung off his every word but he wasn't interested. He'd been to several socials and was clear what he wanted: 'Someone who's 33 or 34. I want children pretty soon so they have to be mature but young enough to not have problems getting pregnant. Back home, women my age are too old for children but women in their 30s don't want to be with a 47-year-old.'

Supply and demand is one reason why these men go Soviet in their spousal hunt. For others, it was more to do with the women being malleable to their needs. I was surprised by how many openly admitted that they wanted to find a pretty, youthful wife who would double up as a housekeeper.

Russell was a 67-year-old retired psychologist from New York. Twice-divorced, he had come to Odessa hoping third-time lucky would bring him a more demure, compliant breed of wife: 'If I were at an event like this back home, I would despise 80 per cent of the women in this room,' he said. 'American women are hideously expectant. They talk about how they want men to inspire them. This wasn't the case 20 years ago: women used to simply ask for a man they can trust, who will help them, who will raise children with them. Now they talk about all this self-esteem crap! They want a man to constantly tell them how great they are.'

His voice was full of contempt, but I was thinking,

'Twenty years ago, women in some states of America had only recently been given the legal right to take out loans. They were only given the all-clear to open their own business, keep their own surname or maintain a separate legal residence in the 70s in some states. Sexism and harassment from men was considered part and parcel of life. Men were paid more for the same roles and employers could sack women as soon as they became pregnant or were judged as having lost their looks. If he wants a wife to live by those cultural mores, he certainly won't find one in New York. And yes, darn right I want a man to inspire me! Otherwise, what's the point?'

'Feminism has gone too far,' Russell continued. 'You women have fought for all these things but now you don't know what you want as a gender. On the one hand, women can't stand men who are assertive. On the other, they don't respect men who aren't. Women here are simple but emotionally strong. They could raise a child on their own in a way that would make most American women crumble. The women here don't fight against us – they are just a delight to be around.'

I couldn't resist asking him if it mattered whether they thought *he* was a delight to be around.

'I know I could give any woman in this room a satisfactory life,' he declared. 'I could buy them everything they'll ever want and more. American women are impossible to make happy. Politically and educationally they are taught to have unrealistic expectations about life. The disparity between how they think life should be and how it is makes them endlessly unhappy. Russian women are more appreciative of men.'

His blinkered ignorance infuriated me. It hadn't occurred

to him that the women he was weighing up for marriage might have a say in it. I thanked him for his time, got up and sat down in front of another middle-class American, only to find he had exactly the same views.

Harry, a 50-year-old from Maine, was – in US-speak – a 'correction officer', which is a prison officer to you and me. Never married, he became a single dad to his two-year-old son after his partner of nine years walked out on them both: 'Western women worry about peripheral things like, what watch do I wear and where are we going on holiday? I hear them say things like "I never cook!" My ex-wife was like that – she would never trim the rose bushes. She'd say, "Can't we just pay someone to do it?" That's not the mentality I want in a woman I want to raise a family with. I'm frugal – I'm not going to pay for something that my able-bodied wife can do! Ukrainian women are born and bred to be wives and their family values are stronger. In America and Europe women want to go to college, get a job and break through glass ceilings. I'm not interested in a woman who is into her professional life, I want a woman who will put me above everything else because that's what I would do for her. I want to come home to a wife in a rocking chair with a baby in her arms and a big smile. It's a small thing, but it means a lot to me.'

'But Harry,' I said. 'Haven't you ever met a woman who simply knocked your socks off because of her captivating intelligence or her awe-inspiring achievements or a great show of strength of character or admirable capability for her job, or her unique creativity, passion and energy? Haven't you ever been mesmerised by a woman like that?'

But he didn't seem remotely affected by my question: 'I do admire those things but ambition would be a deal breaker if it distracted her away from raising a family,' he replied somewhat woodenly.

If I had any remaining faith in the fairytale of ebullient, fulfilling storybook love, these men shattered it. Ambition, independence and dynamism – traits I've always considered attractive – were deal breakers among these men. Never mind love and spiritual connectivity, they just wanted a doormat with a vagina.

For Brandon, 59, divorced for eight years after a 16-year marriage, ambition, independence and individuality were more than deal breakers, they were abhorrent: 'In Europe we've gone from a patriarchal society to a matriarchal society in 20 years,' he argued. 'You women are running the show. Men don't feel respected anymore. Look at sitcoms – a man looking for a date is portrayed as the bumbling idiot. Men and women compete against each other. But I come here and the women are feminine and I find that the more feminine a girl is, the more masculine a man becomes.'

Brandon wasn't looking for anyone to have more children with but he was clear that he wanted to find someone he could take back to the UK to live with him in a stable relationship. 'I'm looking for a soul mate,' he clarified.

Ironically almost every man I spoke to wanted to find a 'soul mate'. I'd catch them in the hotel bar at the end of the day gossiping like girls about 'chemistry levels' and 'feeling a connection'. Yet their idea of what constituted a soul mate was entirely pragmatic. It depended on her willingness to settle down, how easily she might be tamed and how quickly she could learn English.

Raymond, a divorcé from the Midlands, had no qualms about a relationship being more important than the person it is with. He had been married for 17 years before his divorce, four years ago. 'I loved being married,' he said nostalgically. 'I loved having the same face to come home to. I want that again – I like familiarity. I dated a doctor for a year. We got to the stage where we were discussing marriage and even looked at houses together. Her children have some behavioural issues and one day my son said he didn't like going to their house because he didn't like her son. That was it for me. The next day I met her for coffee and you know, had a conversation.'

It sounded heartwrenching. 'But if you were in love with her?' I protested, 'How could you just discard her? You didn't have to live together.'

'No,' he replied firmly. 'If I'm with someone I don't want a twice-a-week thing, always worrying about getting babysitters. I want to live with someone. What's the point of loving someone if you can't have all of them?'

Clearly Raymond preferred the idea of waking up next to someone he hasn't met yet – an idealised stranger – seven days a week rather than waking up beside someone he truly loves twice a week. Pragmatics over romance, needs over desire.

I asked some of the men whether they worried that their prospective Ukrainian brides might be educationally inferior and culturally less experienced. Most of the men had, after all, lived affluent lives, with lots of travel and high-flying careers. 'Just because we've had different lives, doesn't mean we can't love each other,' said one man. 'Perhaps we both like chocolate ice-cream or we both like sci-fi movies. Love – real love – builds up through shared experiences and that's what cements you together.'

And what about that small thing called language? Away from the plentiful interpreters on hand at the Palladium nightclub, it might be hard to cement love. But the men weren't remotely concerned. One told me confidently that a woman could easily learn English within three months if she put her mind to it. Another shrugged: 'A soul mate is a soul mate, I can't request God sends me one with a specific tongue.'

Despite the readily available supply of marriage-minded women, the majority of men had returned to Odessa again and again. It was Harry's fourth romance tour, Brandon's second, Russell's third and Richard had even got engaged to one girl but had a change of heart three months later. That was four years ago and he had been back nearly every year since. I wondered whether the choice itself could be addictive – a little like Internet daters who can't stop logging on and browsing in case there's someone even more marvellous, whom they just haven't met yet.

Whatever the reason, their dithering is certainly good business for Ukraine. Odessa has become a booming hub for marriage tourism. If you're single, female and under 30 in that city, you join a local marriage agency. Signs like 'Catch Your Match', 'Veronikah', 'Amazing Ladies' and 'Odessa Judies' can be seen on every other street. It's impossible to count how many agencies there are because they constantly open, close and change names, but locals estimate there are around 70 agencies in Odessa alone.

The agencies feed the girls' profiles into larger dating websites like AnastasiaDate.com, which serves as an international dating portal containing 27,000 profiles from 17 countries across former Soviet states, Latin America and parts of Asia. Membership of AnastasiaDate.com is free for both women and men, but men have to pay to send messages or to use the site's chat software. Each message costs around

£5 – less if they buy message credits in bulk. The site then passes on a percentage of the fees to the marriage agency providing that girl's profile. So the more girls an agency has on its books, the more money it is likely to make. Some agencies actively scout for single girls.

It's a megabucks industry. Harry, for instance, spends £250 every month for 1,000 'credits'. That gives him 40 messages or 1,000 minutes of chat time plus his yearly 'romance tours' at £3,000 each. At the time of writing there are nearly one million male members of AnastasiaDate.com, which gives a perspective into the price some men are willing to pay to find a mate.

* * *

If, like me, you found the men's words shallow, infuriating even, it's only because we are conditioned so deeply to think that long-term relationships should be based on true love, shared values and psychic synchronicity. That's our fairytale upbringing again. But their version of compatibility is no different to what both sexes believed before the marital love revolution of the eighteenth century. And judging from the women, they have equally self-serving reasons for joining the international dating market.

The first woman I managed to speak to was Irena, 23. I spotted her sitting alone on a round table, running her fingers through her blonde hair, seemingly waiting for a man to approach. She was in her final year of university, studying biology. She'd been with a local marriage agency for three years and was one of the most popular girls on AnastasiaDate.com, thanks to a promotion banner on her profile signposting her as winner of last year's beauty pageant, hosted at a social event such as this. Irena had been on around 20 dates, one of whom took her to his home in Boston.

'I want to get married, I want to meet someone serious. I want to move to the USA and live there,' she said when I asked why she had joined the agency. 'I used to work for one of the agencies and I saw my manager marry one very popular client. She is now living in Germany and they are very rich. He has a helicopter path [sic] on his roof – she is very happy now.'

That is how all the women envisioned happiness – a foreign husband with purchasing power. 'In Ukraine, guys are lazy,' continued Irena. 'They want women to work and support them – that's why the girls want to move.'

I heard similar complaints from every woman. They all seemed to despise their native men and idealise their Western counterparts. Americans, Britons and Europeans were 'more gentle', 'more responsible', 'more interesting', 'more romantic', 'positive', 'kind', 'had manners', 'were good fathers'. Russian men were 'possessive, controlling, non-communicative, aggressive' and they all 'drink too much vodka'.

I asked Irena why she thought Ukrainian men didn't try harder. Surely they feared their apparent insouciance would drive their native women into the arms of foreigners? 'They don't care, they are not looking for a wife – they just like to drink. Some say, "I'll be the best for you, I will work hard for you." Then after you are married they say they don't want to get a job,' was her reply.

Many women had stories of violent exes, like Ekaterina, a 21-year-old manicurist. She had recently split up with an abusive Russian boyfriend. This was her first social event and she told me excitedly that she already had two dates set up later that afternoon and evening, one with an Australian: 'He's a very interesting man with a good sense of humour and not boring. Foreign men are more interesting and more modest – they appreciate women more. Our men don't care about women – they just care about sex.'

It's not just the chivalry that draws the women. The prospect of marriage itself is a big incentive: becoming a wife in Ukraine brings status. 'It's our sole purpose in life,' said Natalia, a 26-year-old retail assistant, proudly. Natalia had a mane of golden blonde curls and was dressed in a tight red Lycra dress and huge clunky heels, which looked too big for her. 'I want to create a family more than anything and I want a good man to do this with. The men at this social are serious about a family because they have flown thousands of miles to find a wife, the men in our country are not serious.'

Natalia's friend, a moody-looking creature with braided hair, each strand dyed a different colour and wearing a jingle-jangle of bracelets, added to this through a translator: 'The man should be the head of the family. If there is not enough money from a husband's job the woman should work too, but nothing too hard. This is because you should remain interesting to your man. If a man comes home after a hard day, he wants a nice environment. The woman should provide a shoulder for the man, good food, maybe a massage. If a woman has also had a hard day and wants to talk about her day, this is not interesting. This creates a not interesting environment for her man.'

I asked Natalia and her friend whether they would still want marriage if money was no object; if they had highflying careers and independence. Their response missed the point but they reflected just how deeply they have internalised their roles. 'I would like to work but I would not take over the man's role,' said Natalia. 'If the man is not as strong as the woman in nature, then the woman should pretend there are things she cannot deal with to make the man feel better. Women who don't pretend to be dependent in marriage, they will fail.'

Her friend insightfully added, through the same stilted interpreter: 'If women are successful and have their own money and see the world, they will find it hard to meet their soul mate. These types of women will always see a man's faults. She will raise her expectations to a level where she will no longer need any man.'

The characteristics to which Western women aspire, in the belief that it makes them more attractive, are the exact ones that these Ukrainian women repress. Who's to say either side is right? Both are playing up to a female stereotype as set by their respective countries' vogues.

When it comes to the male stereotype of attraction, physical attraction barely gets a look-in. I asked several women what they thought of the men physically since it was hard to ignore how much older, greyer and pot-bellied they were compared to their own youthful and immaculate selves. They were obviously expecting this question because they had well-rehearsed lines: 'The belly doesn't matter, it's what's inside,' said one. 'I was brought up to believe every-one is beautiful. I find one thing that is special and that is what I focus on,' was another girl's defence. 'If I find someone has a rich inner world, I find something in their face I like,' went another 22-year-old's vignette.

A lot of the girls had already been involved with men from past romance tours but I never heard one woman talk about specific qualities she loved about her ex-suitor. All of their excitement and enthusiasm came from the reverence of performing wifely duties, dedicating herself to her marriage and raising a family. Not once did any girl single out a man and say, 'Wow, I want to try my luck with him!' Nor did they hint that someone had captured their attention or made them laugh. Shakespeare and Austen would have had a hard time construing any love stories out of an Odessa Palladium nightclub social.

But do you blame them? Had I lived in this freezing city and earned £230 a month with few career opportunities, an unforgiving social pressure to marry despite a shortage of local men, I too would accept a pot-bellied 60-year-old who could provide a nice home in a pleasant American suburb with a car and something in the fridge other than pickled cabbage.

I refer again to sociologist Catherine Hakim's male sex deficit theory. Women's beauty, charm, femininity and sexuality have value because men desire them and because they are more responsive to visual stimuli and women's appearance. Savvy women understand this and use it to their advantage. What Hakim calls 'erotic capital' gives women power both in relationships and in everyday social interaction. For instance, a woman knows that when she's in a nice dress and heels, more men hold doors open for her. Or if she flashes a smile to the man in IT, she'll get her computer fixed sooner. The more overtly she ramps up her feminine charms, the more immediate the rewards. (Hakim in fact wonders why feminism didn't 'champion femininity rather than try to abolish it' and is surprised that no radical thinkers have encouraged women to exploit men, just as men have women.) Blondie singer Deborah Harry summed this up nicely too when she was asked what she thinks of critics who've accused her of 'exploiting her sexuality'. She told Radio 4's *Woman's Hour*: 'I think it's obvious that it was a necessity.'

So the women on the books of Ukrainian marriage agencies are merely using their appearance and youth as leverage to get away from this bankrupt, sexist, freezing-cold industrial town. They are no different to some of the mistresses and paramours we met earlier in Chapter 11. But what happens once they are away from Odessa? Are these pragmatic arrangements a recipe for disaster or do they fare better than those based on genuine romantic love?

For Valya, 30, who now lives in Germany, it didn't work at all. At 19 she had just secured her first full-time job as a junior customs officer on a salary of around £100 per month. She joined a local marriage agency and within six months was engaged to a German. 'When I joined the agency I thought, "Can it really be true that you can feel the same mentality as someone from abroad?" But then I fell in love. He was not so handsome, but he was very good to me. He was 16 years older and I looked up to him. He had seen the world, been to university, had a good job... I only knew Ukrainian men from my town of Nikolai and he was much more interesting.'

After their engagement, it took Valya and her fiancé another year to arrange her visa, during which they visited each other frequently. 'We had never lived together and we hadn't talked about when we would start a family or how we would bring up our children. I presumed that it would happen one day but not yet. I imagined that I would move in with him in his big house in Germany and we would live a few years together, getting to know each other. I would make friends, learn German, be a good wife and we would start a family soon.

'We got married in a small registry office and that very night he said that he wanted to have five children and he wanted to start straight away; he wanted one every year. I told him I didn't want a baby every year, I told him I still wanted to be a lady and look after myself and my body. He became angry and said I was young and I should have children while I was healthy and while I could recover. I cried when he shouted because he had never raised his voice at me before. Then he calmed down and persuaded me that the more children we had, the closer we would be as a family and the more friends I would make because I would get to know all our children's parents.

'After that I kept thinking maybe I was a bad wife for not wanting five children. I kept asking myself: "Do I really want to be a mother and wife, or does everyone else tell me I want this?" My conscious wish was that I wanted to be married and have children but I was trying to understand if this was my subconscious wish too. Because my husband was older and came from a country full of cleverer and more cultured people, I always thought he was right but this time I thought maybe he is not right.

'I started to question my decision to move to Germany. It was isolating. I spoke little German and although his friends' wives and girlfriends were friendly, they were older and they already had children. I became homesick and I craved my own language.'

Valya gave birth to her first child a year after they married. Her husband paid for her mother to fly to Germany to see her. 'I was miserable and crying. My mother kept telling me that I have a good life – I had a husband who was making good money and looking after me and I should stay in Germany.' Valya did stay for another four years and had one more child but two years later she could no longer bear her husband and they divorced. She stayed in Germany because she wanted better opportunities for her daughters than she had had in Ukraine.

'Marrying a foreigner is a pipe dream for women in Russia and Ukraine,' she reflected. 'We have no other way into a nice life, to reach goals, to have children. Many of my friends are in America, they are married and happy. For others it did not work and they have gone back to their country. I tell my girls to make their own life, not to rely on any husband. They will be lucky – they will grow up in Western Europe. They do not have to look to a husband.'

For Toby, 57, and Yana, 31, a mail-order marriage worked out accordantly. Five years ago, Toby signed up to a foreign dating website called UkraineDate.com through frustration with his love life at home. He had divorced his first wife 15 years previously and hadn't had a full-time partner since. His job as a singer regularly took him away on cruise ships for weeks at a time and he liked the idea of having someone at home waiting for him: 'I've always liked to be with someone, I don't like being single. After my divorce I went from one girl to the next. Sometimes they moved in, then they moved out again. I decided to take time out and I was on my own for six months but it's a lonely life when you're touring. There's nothing better than stepping off a flight after weeks away and being able to ring someone. I wanted someone to come home to, I wanted to love someone – something long-term.

'The attraction for me about using an international site was that the girls were younger and more open-minded. There are lots of single people at home – widows and divorced women. I went on lots of Internet dates here but it just wasn't there. When they found out I was an entertainer, women would be impressed by it because it's a bit different and that's all they wanted to talk about. I couldn't help thinking that perhaps they only like me for that reason. On international sites the girls aren't fazed by what I do – I'm different anyway because I'm an English man.'

When Toby first joined the website, he was bombarded with messages: 'I couldn't see the wood for the trees. When you first join, you get contacted by around 20 or 30 girls. Initially you don't have to pay to read them – but that's how they hook you in. You start to learn more and more about each girl, so you get kind of addicted. After so long you have to pay to continue to send messages but by then you can't stop.'

Toby paid the hefty fees for the messenger software so he could chat to Yana nearly every day for two months. The sites have sophisticated software and screening programmes to catch out members who attempt to spell out private emails, phone numbers or Skype IDs, which would allow them to talk more cheaply. Eventually he arranged a trip to Yana's hometown of Donetsk to meet her and her seven-year-old daughter from a relationship with a Ukrainian man.

Why he sparked up a relationship and ended up marrying Yana and none of the other hundreds of beauties who pinged him messages was down to that magic word again: pragmatics. 'It all came down to the communication,' Toby reasoned. 'I'd email and she'd email back straight away – she was keen and efficient, the other girls were flaky. Once you find somebody you like and you contact them regularly, you feel you are building something. So I thought, "I'll nurture this."

'I was her first date and she was my first date – that's very rare apparently. On the flight over, I spoke to other men travelling for the same reasons as me. They had set up dates with four or five girls on one trip. The agencies recommend you do that – if one doesn't work out, they can shrug and say, "I have someone else lined up for you." But I couldn't do that. I had done my groundwork with Yana and if it didn't work, I'd get the next flight back. Men who go to socials to pick from a tribe of women are essentially just paying for numbers. I'd taken the time to get to know Yana and build trust.'

So, I asked Toby, could he have forged a marriage with any pretty girl who happened to be efficient, responsive and appeared to be genuine?

'Yes,' he admitted. 'If I'd met someone else equally serious, I would have married her. If I'm honest, every girl I hit on was pretty but always at the back of my mind when I started out was the thought, "Why does one of these beautiful girls want to be with me?" On the plane over, I was thinking, "How do I know the girl I am about to meet doesn't just want a passport or is after my money?" They are worried about us, too – they are warned that foreign men come over, woo them, say they love them and then bring them to their country and put them in the prostitution business. So you have to work to build trust from both sides.

'When I met someone who did seem genuine and serious, I pursued her. I took time to see her around her family and friends in her natural surroundings. She was religious and went to church. I'm not religious but that mattered because it indicated she was honest.'

When I spoke to Yana – separately – she too said that focus was the recipe for success: 'When I joined the site I was looking for a husband and a family: Toby was that. When we talked, I thought straight away he is serious – he wanted to know everything about me. Some men just ask what you do and that's it. But Toby was asking me many questions, like what I did today, what I plan for the future, what I dream about. When a man asks lots of questions, a woman knows he is serious. When I met him I could see how he was a nice person with a good heart. I knew that this was my husband of the future. I thought, "I will not let him go, I will work very hard at this." He didn't just come to have fun or have sex, or spend money and show off – he came to look for a wife.'

On Toby's first visit he and Yana spent 10 days together. When he left, he set her up with a laptop, Skype account and paid for her to have English lessons so they could keep in touch. At the end of his third visit he proposed and they married just six months after he first initiated Internet contact. The visa process took several more months, something they both describe as 'a nightmare'. Then Yana and her daughter followed Toby to the Midlands, where they have lived for two years.

'People think finding a wife abroad is the easy route, but it's actually harder,' Toby explained. 'You can't just go over once and marry a girl, I went six or seven times. It's easy in this country to find a girl and get married and if it doesn't work, get a divorce. But when you've found a girl in a different country, bought several flights to see her, paid for her to learn your language, dragged her away from her family to a country she's never been to with her young daughter, who's had to leave all her friends too, it's a bigger commitment: it's a moral commitment.

'In the early days when I was going to Ukraine regularly,

people would say, "But what if it doesn't last?" But I could marry a girl who lives in my street and that may not last. The fact that we put so much effort into being together means I'm less likely to stray and so is she. It was a lovely feeling when she first moved in – I loved showing someone our country, the history, where we live and our dog. It was exciting. I was well aware that she left her family and friends so I made an extra effort to help her settle. We decorated the spare bedroom for her daughter – she'd never had her own room so that was special for her.

'Yana has her moments where she says, "I want to go back to Ukraine!" She misses her friends and family. At night she is forever on Skype or she is streaming films in Russian. She doesn't go out because she has no friends so I do worry about her. I went away for five weeks working on a cruise and when I came back, boy, was she depressed! She doesn't drive so she had been cocooned at home with her daughter for all that time. But I say, "We've done so much to be together, divorce is not part of our vocabulary."'

Toby and Yana's life now is remarkably normal. They live like any other married couple; they enjoy the cinema and long walks, and go on holiday once a year. On weekends he plays football with his two sons from his previous marriage and she goes swimming with her daughter. 'It's as if she's always been with me,' Toby says happily. Their marriage is shaped on the simple pleasures of companionship. By Toby's own admission he could have married any of the girls with shared values but they had also grown to love each other. They'd almost manufactured their love, which may not appeal to romance chasers, but the recipe was exactly right for them. Their relationship is another example of how relationships almost always balance out cost and worth. For

Yana and Toby their huge investments, both financial and personal, were well worth it.

Wooing his Russian bride cost Toby nearly £15k once he'd accounted for seven return flights, Yana's visa and his message fees to the marriage agencies. Every year he now pays to send her home for a month and pays the costs of bringing up her daughter. So does that bother him? 'I'm left with significantly less disposable income than when I was living as a carefree Don Juan flitting between women, but that isn't what I wanted. Money doesn't bother me. We come into this world with no money and we leave with no money. I put mine to the best possible use!' he laughed.

Yana also considers her life sacrifices small change: 'I was scared about moving to England. I hadn't even seen where I would live, only in a photo, but I said to myself, I have to trust my husband and go. When I arrived, I hardly spoke English and I had no friends around me. For six months I couldn't go anywhere without my husband with me. I couldn't ask for things in shops, I felt guilty about moving my daughter out of her school to a country where she cannot understand anyone. Now she is fluent – far more than me. I was concerned that my own daughter would grow up more English than Russian but I made my decision to come here and it was worth it. In my last relationship with the father of my daughter, he did not care for her. He never asked how I was feeling and he never called to say "Happy Birthday" and things like that. Now I have someone who is there for me and that makes me very happy.'

CHAPTER 15

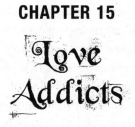

Love
Addicts

@f all this focus on pragmatic love has left you
despondent, I'm now going to demonstrate what
happens when you base your relationships on the more
unreliable sentiments of romantic love and passion. I warn
you, it's not like they say it is in the fairytales.

If you want a shortcut to this chapter, watch the film
Crazy Love. It's based on a true story, which started in
the 1950s after New York lawyer Bert Pugach started to date
his younger lover, Linda Riss. Bert became well and truly
besotted with her, despite being already married. Eventually
Linda gave up hope that he'd ever leave his wife and so she
found her own husband-to-be. On finding out she was
engaged, Bert flipped and hired thugs to blind her. After two
decades in prison and a divorce, he was still as obsessively in
love with her as ever: they eventually married.

According to some reports, a policewoman assigned to
guard Linda while Burt awaited trial persuaded her to marry
him. She apparently told her that if she didn't get back with

him, she might end up old and alone. Better to be with a thug, eh? We may cringe at this but for someone addicted to love, even bad love is better than none. Linda was as much a love addict as her crazy, frenzied lover Bert.

Love addiction is much less talked about than its anti-matter 'commitment-phobia' but it's taken far more seriously, at least within the self-help world and among *au current* psychologists. And yes, the affliction is just as messy as Robert Palmer made it sound in the lyrics to his 1980s hit, 'Addicted to Love'.

For decades, love addiction has been well documented in the States (where else, I hear you say, than a country where you can get therapy for stubbing your toe?). But in the last 10 years, it's slowly made its way onto the menus of European therapists too and increasingly high-profile treatment programmes are cropping up.

Most well known is a 12-step counter-addiction programme, Sex and Love Addicts Anonymous (SLAA) set up in the 1970s by a member of Alcoholics Anonymous in Boston who could not stay faithful to his wife, even though he loved her. He noticed a correlation between his alcoholism and his compulsion for romantic and sexual fixes so he adapted the 12-step recovery programme. There were plenty of people who could relate to this because his programme soon caught on and there are now 16,000 members of SLAA, with meetings in 43 different countries. Like alcoholics, love addicts go to meetings to learn to be 'sober'. That is, they try to live without their addiction – relationships.

Eager to find out more about this condition, I bravely rocked up to a few SLAA meetings in London. I was particularly nervous about this latest covert operation. Not only was I expecting a room filled with the negative energies of heartbreak and desperation, what would my 'love addiction' cover story be? I'm a commitment-phobe at a meeting for commitment *addicts*! Not MI5's choice of secret agent, for sure.

As with all my secret pilgrimages, I try to dig deep for a personal reason why I want to find out about a certain culture or community. That way I attend not as a curious bystander but as a participant. As I read about love addiction, I learned that there is one type who gets hooked on the romance: they never stay in a long-term relationship because they're constantly chasing the butterfly feeling of new love. So actually, perhaps I wasn't so immune after all. This in itself was enough to justify my trip.

There were around 25 in the first SLAA meeting I attended, a 60–40 split of the sexes. Most of the women looked under 40, many in their 20s with a fresh-faced college graduate look about them. As I scurried in, I detected laughter and educated accents. They seemed a lively and good-looking crowd. Take away the church hall meeting room and the choir practice above us and these were the sort of faces you'd expect to meet at any half-decent bar or young office. Most had appeared in work clothes for the 6.30 p.m. start.

There were exchanges of: 'How have you been this week?' 'Emotionally up and down but sticking to the programme'. Or: 'Been a while?' 'Yeah, I felt good. Didn't think I needed the meetings but some bad stuff has happened and I'm on that spiral again'.

Twelve-step fellowships follow a rigid format, beginning with a moment's silence and then a reading of what is known as a 'serenity prayer'. This is followed by a preamble of what

LOVE ADDICTS

Sex and Love Addicts Anonymous is and its aim (to counter the destructive consequences of sex and love addiction). Then there's a definition of whatever theme is being discussed in that particular session. In this case it was 'emotional anorexia' – when sufferers withhold themselves from the nurturing properties of love because they are scared of intimacy. Afterwards one person volunteers to 'chair'. This means they take 15 minutes to share their story and their recovery progress with the group. The chair on this occasion was Mick, a floppy-haired blond in his mid-40s, who looked like a surfer. When he announced that he would be speaking, everyone chorused with, 'Thanks, Mick'. Someone called Ed was nominated to keep time and after every five minutes, he'd put one finger up, to which Mick would respond, 'Thanks, Ed'.

Mick told the group about a childhood overshadowed by his parents' rows and how it had driven him to spend all his time out of the house. Through boredom he started to drink as a teenager. When the novelty faded, drinking turned to drug taking and then it was women and sex. Before he knew it, he had become a young adult with no prospects, addicted to booze, drugs and prostitutes.

'I used booze, drugs and sex as a way to feel something – it was the only way actually. I stayed in that bubble for 30 years. There was lots of sex, lots of one-night stands, prostitutes. There was never any emotion in any of the encounters, but at least there was something there, something to feel. With some of the women it was just sex. With others I'd convince myself there was a connection and I'd create this huge fantasy around them. I'd imagine how I might see them again and maybe make something of us but there was never anything there, of course.

'I did have relationships but I always sabotaged them – I couldn't deal with the emotional reality when a girl wanted to get close. Everything I did was total self-destruct. I did some crazy things, truly crazy. I had lots of crashes because of the drugs and then I'd drink and seek sex to feel something again. It was a cycle.'

Because SLAA meetings are deeply personal events, I have represented only snippets of Mick's and other members' stories. The meetings make clear that they provide an environment for people to heal and offload their stories free from judgement. As with all addiction fellowship programmes – Alcoholics Anonymous, Narcotics Anonymous and Gamblers Anonymous – there is a firm rule that anything within the walls of the meetings stays there and they make a point of never seeking publicity. SLAA is not interested in profit, nor affiliated to any other organisation, cause or movement but concerned only with helping people. For that reason, what I've reported below about these meetings is only intended to reflect a taste of the different experiences of love and sex addiction. Those whose stories I have told in greater detail are because I later gained their permission to do so.

Mick's speech was rounded off with a chorus of 'Thanks, Mick'. Then each circle member had a three-minute opportunity to respond. Some picked up on a part of Mick's chair that had resonated with them. Others soliloquised, using their three minutes to verbalise streams of consciousness reflecting their own recovery status and particular struggles that week. Each started with, 'Thanks for your chair, Mick', followed by their name and a declaration as to whether they were a sex addict, love addict, fantasy addict or a combination of all three. Ed kept up the clock-watching, raising his hand at every 60-second point, to which the speaker would acknowledge, 'Thanks, Ed'.

One woman in her mid-thirties with thick, black curly hair and snow-white skin, told how she had never had the confidence to be single, but thanks to the programme she was learning to trust herself more. 'I've always felt that I needed to go to someone else for the answer – in a work situation, with friends, boyfriends. But I always had the answers inside of me all the time. Withdrawal has been hard but I feel free now because I'm learning to be on my own. I'm not desperately leaning on someone as I have my whole life – I feel I have more dignity now.'

Another man, who introduced himself to me at the end after spotting I was a newcomer, had only been practising the Twelve Steps Program for six weeks. His last relationship ended two years previously but he had still not recovered from the heartbreak. 'I was on the floor for 12 months,' he told me. 'I couldn't do anything – I was totally knocked out, my business suffered. I lost touch with friends. I went feral almost, not showering or bothering with anything. I couldn't think for myself any more – I had become dependent on her for my whole sense of self-worth. When we were together, there were lots of things I didn't like about her behaviour and conversationally we never went that deep, but I was addicted to knowing that I had a girlfriend. I needed to wake up and see someone sleeping beside me to feel OK. I think I needed a girlfriend as a distraction from the other realities in my life – that my business wasn't going well, that I'd lost certain friends, that my life wasn't how I wanted it.

'Things are going well for me now,' he continued. 'I actually managed to go on a date last week – the first time since going sober. She was perfectly nice. But I called her today and already I could feel myself getting hooked in. I could feel myself thinking, "This could be the start of a relationship." I was building things up in my head, galloping ahead, making plans around her; that's exactly what I did in my last relationship. I lose myself in relationships. So I ended the phone call before I started to go down that road. I don't think I'm ready yet to date.'

Then an American girl of around 25 used her three minutes to compare Mick's turbulent childhood with her own: 'My father is a horrible man – he cut me off after years of being physically abusive. But despite the bad he's done, cutting me off was the most painful thing. I would prefer to have him in my life and working on his problems rather than not in my life. In the same way I've always felt I'd rather have an abusive partner in my life working on things that aren't right, rather than leaving my life altogether. Especially if there are parts of them I like and we have history together.'

Her comments made me think of Gemma, the glamorous single mum we met in Chapter One. Gemma was this girl's antithesis. She had remained single simply because she wouldn't stick with a relationship that wasn't perfect. Of course it meant she had never found a full-time partner, but she considered it felicitous to her life, not a cause for sorrow.

Now, I don't wish to make huge generalisations simply from a few contrasting case studies but I can't help clocking this as another match point for singledom. Neither Gemma nor any of the other contented singletons mentioned in earlier chapters had ever found their ruthless approach to love had landed them in group therapy. I'm not saying chasing love will always lead to mental breakdown but if I had to choose between being obsessed about my relationships or being a love cynic, I'd say the latter was a safer bet.

If you don't believe me, Nina provides an exemplary case study of how love addiction can rule one's life. As a 32-year-old financial consultant, she appears to have it all. She has a high-powered job in the financial services sector, which affords her a swish apartment, luxury holidays, a fine wardrobe and the means to pursue her expensive weekend hobby of sailing. She's athletic, with exotic features from her Italian family and a bright personality but she concedes underneath it all she feels constant romantic longing. It isn't that she can't find a boyfriend; she has plenty of offers but she can't stop herself from going for unavailable men. Whenever a decent type takes interest, she becomes bored or picks fault.

'I think I am addicted to the feeling of longing,' Nina began. She had a lovely smile and huge, slightly startled eyes. 'I thrive on the torment of dreaming about someone I can't have – of idolising someone. I've done it all my life. It's like I need the pain of wanting something; it's like I try to inflict extremities of emotion on myself. It's somehow purging. I deliberately torment myself by wanting some man I can't have. I joke to myself that I must be like Damien Hirst – I deliberately deprive myself of something to enhance the sensation.

'As a teenager I started experiencing desperate obsessions with men I couldn't have – my dad's friend or a teacher. There has nearly always been a figure in my life that I can't get out of my head. But it never goes on from there: because they are married, or they are in a foreign country or a position of authority. Or they are in another way inappropriate.

'I don't know if I subconsciously seek these men out –

believing them to be "safer" than a single man, who is at risk of getting too close. Or whether they are attracted to me because I seem safely non-demanding. I work long hours and sail on weekends so I'm hardly going to get clingy. Or is it more sinister and I am attracted to taken men because I see them as a challenge? "He's married and I got him into bed!" – I don't think that's the case; I hope not. I never feel a sense of triumph in any of my romantic conquests but it has to be more than coincidence why I only like unavailable men. Why I can't just fall for someone who asks me out at a party or something, I do not know. It's as if I need to feel this intense sense of craving in order to feel that there is anything in it.'

When I met Nina she was two years into an affair with a married man. Desperately aware of how destructive it was, she couldn't walk away. They worked for different companies but regularly attended the same training centre. She insisted that when the affair began, she didn't want anything more that the excitement of a clandestine affair but the more elusive he was, the more addicted she became.

Nina told me story after story of how he had let her down. Many times she vowed to call it off but she kept running back. She couldn't free herself from her addiction and every time she bumped into him on training days, he'd leap back into her thoughts. 'It was a friend who made me realise that I was addicted to the relationship. She said to me, "How flattering it is for him to have a girl like you hanging on his every word. If you stay with him, you've got so much more to lose than him." I told her that he had more to lose because he was risking his family by having an affair, and she said, "No, you've got more to lose. He's had his family – you have your heart to lose, your youth and your fertility!"

'It hit me then that I couldn't end it, even if I wanted to. I knew that the only way I could get him out of my head was if I got obsessed with someone else. I don't want to be like this anymore, I want to fancy someone in a healthy way so that it doesn't take over my life. My whole life feels like it's been one never-ending pursuit of the unattainable.'

* * *

Around a decade after SLAA was set up, love addiction was propelled into popular consciousness after a self-help book called *Women Who Love Too Much* by psychologist Robin Norwood became a bestseller. It was based on interviews with hundreds of women who had consulted her because relationship obsession was taking over their lives. (Norwood initially believed love addiction affected mainly women but the consensus now is that men and women are equally prone to addictive relationship patterns.)

Since then many more writers and psychological professionals have delved into the subject and spawned various theories and definitions. One such theory was put forward by Brenda Schaeffer, a Minnesota-based psychologist, in *Is It Love or Is It an Addiction?* Schaeffer said that love and relationship addiction was on a par with alcohol, tobacco or drug addiction because the cravings go along the same neuropathway for satiation. She claimed that after a break-up people experience a withdrawal from all the feel-good chemicals that the person they've left behind used to elicit in them.

She was on the right lines. Since Schaeffer's book, recent scientists have identified such a chemical. Already we know about the role of dopamine and noradrenalin in early romantic love, now there's interest in a more specific chemical – phenylethylamine, or PEA – which is known as dopamine's little helper, because it's the thing that helps us release dopamine and all the feel-good things that go with it.

PEA makes the heart beat faster and causes feelings of euphoria. We emit it after strenuous exercise, when we see someone we fancy or while watching an arousing movie. Also the organic compound found in chocolate, it's being researched as a potential treatment for depression, ADHD and even obesity because it suppresses appetite (which would perhaps explain the popular wisdom that love makes you go off your food). The theory now is that love addicts get hooked on the PEA in their system and following withdrawal, it's bad news.

One of the most quoted counsellors on love addiction is Susan Peabody. A decade ago she herself went through the Twelve Steps Program, then set up her own support group in California called LAA. It's like SLAA without the sex because she believes that love addiction and sex addiction shouldn't be lumped together.

'I wanted to give love addicts a home,' she explained. 'A love addict just won't get any good from being in a room full of compulsive masturbators or paedophiles – they are totally different conditions. A sex addict seeks sexual experiences in isolation – pornography, masturbation, prostitutes – they'll avoid any sort of bonding. If you bond even a little bit, you're a love addict. Tiger Woods was portrayed as a sex addict, but because he saw some of those women more than once, I'd say he was more of a romance addict.'

The 'romance addict' is one of Peabody's five types of love addict, which have become the most commonly referenced explanation in popular literature on the subject. Brace yourself because the five breeds of love addict make for a flighty bunch indeed, and given how crazy we all get about love occasionally, you may be in danger of some hypo-chondriac self-diagnosis – I certainly was.

First, there's the obsessed love addict. They will stay obsessed with their partner even if he/she is totally unsuitable, unloving, distant, unavailable, controlling or even abusive.

Then there's the relationship addict, who has the opposite problem. They may no longer be in love with their partner but they can't let go. Sometimes they're so unhappy, their health or happiness may be affected but they are scared of change and afraid of being alone.

Thirdly, there is the narcissistic love addict. They are the mean selfish brutes in the relationship but they can't help it; they can be dominating and controlling and demand their own way. While they come across as aloof or uncaring if you try to leave them, wow! They'll do anything in their power to stop you or get you back, even resorting to stalking or violence.

Peabody's fourth type is the co-dependent love addict, which she believes is the most common. The co-dependent suffers low self-esteem so they try to hold onto the person to whom they are addicted by becoming their caregiver. They will make their partner feel he/she can't live without them so they won't leave them. Often they go for partners in need of 'fixing' such as alcoholics or similarly addictive personalities because it promises the reward of validation if they can be their saving grace.

And finally, there is the avoidant (or ambivalent) love addict. They don't have a hard time letting go, they have a hard time moving forward. Although they desperately crave love, they are scared of intimacy and use various tactics to stay detached emotionally. These are the so-called 'emotional anorexics' mentioned frequently at SLAA meetings. A love avoidant may become a 'torch bearer' and become fixated on someone unavailable. Or they might exhibit their symptoms as a 'saboteur', constantly messing up a relationship as soon as it gets serious. Or, like Tiger Woods, they could be a 'romance addict' – hooked on the honeymoon stage.

Sex addiction was thrust into the media spotlight when Woods was exposed as having affairs with several women, including glamorous nightclub promoter, Rachel Uchitel. He reportedly checked himself into an addiction clinic in Mississippi. The media thought it could only be one thing – 'sex addiction' – and so followed much deliberation as to whether sex addiction is a real condition. For the record, it's not. In the same way that commitment phobia isn't on the DSM (forgive the repetition but that's the diagnostic 'bible' of mental health disorders) but still resonates with many, neither is sex addiction. On the DSM the closest official condition to sex addiction would be hypersexuality – an obsessive urge for sex. But hypersexuality usually occurs as a result of medication or a symptom of other underlying conditions, like bipolar disorder. So the term 'sex addiction' is really just a catchy coinage by media-savvy psychologists, therapists and life coaches to describe behaviour on the eyebrow-raising end of normal.

It's much the same situation with love addiction. The psychiatric profession doesn't acknowledge love addiction per se (so if you committed a crime of passion or killed the person you were addicted to with an axe, this would not stand up in court). But two other items on the DSM come close to it.

The first is erotomania. An erotomaniac has an

unshakeable belief that another person, often a stranger or a celebrity, is in love with them. Convinced their admirer is communicating with them through special glances, signals or even messages through the media, they take it upon themselves to return the affection. They'll send letters and gifts, make phone calls and even turn up at their desired one's home. John Hinckley was thought to suffer from erotomania when he attempted to assassinate Ronald Reagan over his obsession with Jodie Foster.

The other item in the DSM to ring bells with love addiction is attachment disorder (sometimes called Reactive Attachment Disorder or RAD). As the name suggests, someone with attachment disorder has difficulty bonding with people in a healthy way. They find it hard to trust people but once they do, it's hard to let go. Individuals can be controlling and manipulative, anger easily and feel insecure. It's thought to stem from a failure to form loving attachments to caregivers in early childhood and, sadly, the consequence of neglect, abuse or abrupt separation from parents.

Susan Peabody is well aware that the psychiatric profession doesn't recognise love addiction or sex addiction but that doesn't stop her and therapists like her treating it seriously. 'The psychiatric professionals – the ones with the most degrees – consider love addiction to be psychobabble,' she sighs. 'Psychologists and therapists may be less academic but they are on the front line, seeing clients and so they are the ones spotting common themes and behaviour that are affecting many people's lives. Whatever the psychiatric community thinks, I get letters from clients saying that I've saved their life.'

She views love addiction as basically the adult version of

attachment disorder. 'If you are a love addict, it's because you didn't get your needs met in childhood,' she says matter-of-factly. 'The love addict develops what I call the hungry heart. They go searching for what they didn't have in childhood and they fixate on anyone who they think can fulfil it. If that person tries to leave, they'll feel separation anxiety – the exact symptoms of attachment disorder.'

So, what I'm sure you are dying to find out is how do we know if we are a besotted love addict, or simply a little excited about a new man/woman in our life? As Dr Helen Fisher said in an earlier chapter, all romantic love is obsessive by its very nature! If we call anyone who can't stop checking their phone for a text from their lover every hour a love addict, surely we're in danger of labelling the whole population psychologically unhinged?

'Basically you know a tree by its fruit,' explains Peabody. 'Everyone experiences emotions during a break-up but the love addict gets attached like Super Glue, so when someone leaves their life, it triggers all their childhood abandonment wounds. They experience age regression, their childhood instincts kick in and tell them they may die if their love object leaves them.

'Addictions are progressions, so there's a fine line to cross. Some people may get close to addictive behaviour and others may go right over it. If you cross the line it's because you are thinking like an addict, acting like an addict. You're obsessed, you can't think of anything else, you are out of control. If you can't go a few hours without speaking to your object of desire then you're an addict. If you have suicidal thoughts after a trial separation, you are an addict.

'If, after the honeymoon period, you start believing that only this person in the world can fulfil you, you're an addict.

LOVE ADDICTS

All people are replaceable. You can fall in love many times but love addicts don't think that way. They think: "I've waited all my life for this person – they are my soul mate, I can't live without them. If they're gone, I want to die."'

* * *

On face value, the so-called 'romance addict' love avoidant could well describe the very relationship values that I've proudly endorsed. As you know, I'm the biggest advocate of the part-time relationship. In the past I have associated romance pretty much with cocktails on tall bar stools and weekends away and very little to do with pushing a trolley around the supermarket. And earlier on in this book, didn't I state that romantic love is the biggest human high of all?

I must admit, at the SLAA meeting I did tick a few boxes on the 'diagnostic questions' I was given. For instance, I haven't had many long relationships – mostly short ones. I tend to have lots of acquaintances but few close friends. I'm always busy, usually doing things on my own. These were some of the alleged telltale symptoms of an avoidant love addict. Perhaps I'm a closet romance addict, I thought, and not a rounded happy singleton after all. Maybe I'm just hiding from love because it's a way to keep the buzz going? And if so, how's that different from being a commitment-phobe? Or are romance addicts/love avoidants simply more derogatory labels for those who dare to opt out of the fairytale? Actually I think it is different. Healthy trepidation about merging your entire life with someone is worlds apart from the deep sense of longing, frustration and drama experienced by real love addicts and avoidants.

Annabel, for instance, whom I also befriended after a

SLAA visit admits that her 'love avoidance and romance addiction' is in danger of ruining her marriage. Having recently got back with her husband after a two-year separation, she turned to SLAA to stop history repeating itself. 'I wasn't the sort of love addict that sits by the phone for hours, waiting for it to ring,' she relayed. 'I was addicted to the buzz of meeting someone new, of sex with someone new, the excitement that they could bring to my life, the fantasy of the potential, what would happen next.'

Annabel and her husband got together in their early 20s and married at 30. He slowly turned from a social to a heavy drinker to an alcoholic. This, she reflected, worked to her advantage because it gave her plenty of opportunities to have guilt-free affairs. 'We were that happy couple you see on Facebook, going to Michelin-starred restaurants every weekend and [on] exotic holidays but the reality was we were really unhappy.

'The whole time I was married, I fantasised about other people. Everywhere I went, I would scan a room for potential. On a train I would know where every man in the carriage, old and young, was sitting. I'd know what man was looking at me and if I found him attractive. It was empowering to know that I was desired and that I could get someone's number, or get someone to meet me or go to bed with me within hours.

'Last summer things got really bad. The fantasies turned into affairs and when my supply of men for flings ran dry, I used websites where people meet for sex. I now know that I did it to escape intimacy with my partner – it was a way of putting things between us. When we divorced, my affairs came out; I used his alcoholism to blame him. I said that he wasn't paying me attention so it drove me to affairs. But he wasn't to blame – I used my affairs as a tool to prevent myself getting too close to him.

'Him being an alcoholic suited me because it made him emotionally unavailable. When he went to AA and got sober, he engaged with me again, asking me questions, gazing at me in a certain way. I couldn't deal with it – I didn't want that level of closeness so I used other ways of pushing him away and that was other people. I now see that for my whole life I've been looking for ways to avoid intimacy. At work I'd always be thinking, how I could arrive or leave so that I wouldn't bump into people or have to go to lunch with people.'

Annabel's 'sobriety' required her to set what are known as 'bottom lines' – things that she vowed not to do. She had to promise herself that she wouldn't fantasise about men, be drawn into emailing men, seek potential in everyone she met or have any unnecessary contact with men. If she had to speak to a male member of staff through her job as a lab technician, she kept it as brief as possible. She chose not to drink during her recovery because even though she's a restrained drinker, it made her 'scan the room'.

'I've come a long way,' she sighed. 'My husband knows I've done the SLAA programme but he doesn't know the extent of my affairs. He says the difference in me is amazing. I never used to let him hug me, I've been like that for 10 years. Now we hug all the time. But whether we can ever have a truly intimate relationship, I don't know. When one person changes in a relationship, it often disrupts the balance. I'm far from settled, but it's nice to be with him and not fantasise about other people.

'I've examined my childhood since coming to these meetings and I now know that my parents didn't have the tools to give me inner confidence and love. When we seek meaningless sex, what we are doing is deriving our need for self-worth and validation from the wrong place. I thought having man after man telling me they desired me would fulfil that, I didn't want them to love me or get close to them – I wanted men to be in awe of me.'

* * *

The roots to hopeless love addiction and all this destructive clinginess may well lie in our childhood experiences but constant cultural reference to the happy-ever-after fairytale doesn't help. One recovering co-dependent love addict called Daisy explicitly blames this for perpetuating her obsession with finding, holding onto and impressing men. Her story is tragicomic. Now 38, she is retraining to become a therapist after a stop-start career as a filmmaker. A pretty, Irish-blooded redhead with limitless energy, boy she could talk! But she was funny and likeable, with a strong sense of self-understanding – the result, she says, of years of therapy.

'Up until my early 30s relationships were really my whole life,' she began. 'Since puberty I thought about men non-stop – I got my sense of self-worth from how many men liked me, relationships gave me a high that was everything to me. It was what made me feel worthwhile and alive. My life was constant highs and lows, which I now see were no different to drug addiction.

'I grew up with a co-dependent mother, who lived her life pleasing men. My grandmother was the same. My two sisters and I were all men crazy and there was vicious competition over boyfriends; there was this belief in our household that if you were single, everyone would think badly of you. I even dated people I didn't like because I felt that if I didn't have a man, I was a loser.

'At age 11, my mother was buying me dishes and things for my bottom drawer. She'd go to car boot sales and come back with second-hand spatulas. I was taught that you grow up and you're a wife; there was never any talk about living your dreams and *maybe* you'll get married. It was always "You must find a man" – that's what you do.

'I had endless, short, quick, fiery, dramatic relationships. I'd fall totally in love straight away, get high from it and then crash – I didn't know that when you meet someone you're allowed to take your time to get to know them. I believed the Hollywood baloney that you meet someone and it's fireworks, and that's love.

'I sabotaged everything for boyfriends. I worked hard to get into film school and then to get my first career break. Finally, I managed to get a meeting with a senior director on a big channel. He was really keen on two of my ideas and all I had to do was write up a more detailed draft. But what did I do? I got involved with a man and I went to Iceland with him. Months went by and I still hadn't sent the director anything. I would always let everything drop when I met a man – the relationship would always come first. I'd be at their house and I'd say, "I must go home and do some work" and they'd say, "Oh, let's do this or that." And I'd stay with them because I thought the relationship was more important than anything I needed to do.

'Their careers wouldn't suffer because I would be helping *them*. One time I dated a guy who owned a bike shop. I went in to get a puncture fixed and the next day we were dating. Within days I was working in his shop because he needed someone to help out. I went into co-dependent mode as I always did. It was a case of: "They'll love me because they'll think I'm wonderful and helpful" – I didn't see a healthy, mutually supportive relationship as an option, everything had to be intense.'

Despite the fact that Daisy always had to be in a relationship, her longest was only six months. 'I'd get them obsessed with me and then I'd run away,' she explained. 'I thought that when you meet a man you have to make him adore you and do everything in your power to get him hooked into you. Once I'd proved to myself I could do that, I'd break up with him and that led to all sorts of drama, like him stalking me or threatening me.

'Here's the strange thing,' she continued thoughtfully. 'I've never actually been dumped, but that's because if there was so much as a sniff that he may dump me, I'd run. I had lots of one-night stands where I wanted more but when it became apparent that they didn't, I'd walk away and pretend I never liked them either. Lots of love addicts are like that – they are so used to escaping their pain their whole life that as soon as they think they may be hurt, they leave. The truth was, with every one-night stand, I wanted to make that man love me and stay with me. If it didn't work out that way, I would lie to my girlfriends about it – I'd make a story up about how he was a loser and I didn't return his call, or that we only kissed even if it was more.

'I got myself a terrible reputation because I slept around. One time during college I visited cousins in America – it was the first time I'd met them, everything was going really well. My cousin and I were getting on like peas in a pod and she took me out for the night. Imagine it – I had just met them, I was staying at their family home having just arrived from England and on my second night, I met a guy and I told my cousin I was going home with him! She was horrified. She had to go home and tell her parents where I'd gone. They didn't even speak to me after that and I had to go home early. I was so ashamed but I couldn't stop myself doing those things.

'I was never happy unless I had someone interested in me. I didn't ever cheat but I overlapped. For example, if I sensed a boyfriend was losing interest, I would find a man to be my best friend and have him waiting in the wings, and then as soon as one relationship ended, I'd jump into the arms of the new one.'

Daisy lived like this until at age 30, a chance conversation with a senior colleague at work caused her to question her relationship patterns. 'I must have been talking about one of the men in my life because this woman said to me in total exasperation, "How often do you think of men?" I thought, "Well, all the time." It was only when she asked me that question that it hit me that it wasn't normal. So I started asking friends how often they think about men and whether they check men out everywhere they go, and when I found that they didn't, it was a shock.

'At around the same time I'd discovered Internet dating and I knew that I was using it in a weird way. I would spend hours on sites chatting to men. I got all these guys liking me and then they'd ask to meet and I just wouldn't bother – I didn't want to meet them, I just wanted to feel I could attract men's attention. I became obsessed with it. I'd tell friends I couldn't meet them because I was busy or working, when really I'd stay at home chatting online with strangers. I started to ask myself, why am I hiding this? Why am I ashamed?'

Between relationships, Daisy was also experiencing bouts

of depression: 'I was using relationships like a drug – I'd make them very intense and get high off them and then when they ended, I'd get real lows.' It was all these things that made her take herself to counselling. During therapy she was encouraged to talk with her mother about her childhood and she learned that in her pre-school years, her mother had repeatedly walked out for several weeks before returning. Daisy hadn't remembered it, but she and her sisters were apparently traumatised.

'I now know why I was forcing all these men to fall in love with me and then leaving them – that's me as a child proving to my mother that I'm lovable and then punishing her for leaving. I was saying, "Ha! I can get your love, but now I'm going to screw you. I'm going to destroy you!" Sometimes, if I really wanted to punish a guy, I'd go back with him late at night, I'd get him all excited and then I'd say, "Oh, I'm leaving now."

'You see, it was never about the sex. It was about knowing that I could have them if I wanted to. One time at sixth-form college my best friend had been telling me how much she was in love with a guy on her course. A few nights later I was drunk in a pub and I met a guy by the same name, on the same course. I was pretty sure it must be him but you know what, I just couldn't resist. I didn't even like him but it was the thrill that he chose me over her – I felt powerful, I was the chosen one.'

Daisy is now full of remorse for her love addictive past. She battles guilt for 'screwing over friends and men for my own feeling of power.' On the recommendation of one therapist she went 'sober' of men and relationships for two years. Bar the odd blip, she is now single and much calmer – 'I can't believe it took therapy to make me realise I love being single. In the last three years I've spent more time on my own than in my whole life put together and I love it.

'But I still have to be conscious of using relationships and men to feel better,' she added. 'I'm sorry to say it, but I believe like drink and drug addictions, it is something you have to work with for life.'

If that's the case, it will certainly keep her in business. Daisy recently started her own 'man detox' programme for women with similar problems. Her mission is to change the culture which she says fuels love addiction: 'As a society we've mistaken addictive ideas of love for what love really is. It's almost become aspirational to have dramatic, draining, difficult relationships because we are taught that love has to hurt to be real.

'We're bombarded with romance books and movies from a young age with this addictive idea of love. We're taught that we'll instantly know when we meet The One. No one tells you that you can spend a lot of time getting to know a guy before you jump in. People think they'll have some epiphany when they meet their soul mate and they'll be on fire for them – but we shouldn't even be looking! We should be focusing entirely on our own path, living our life on our own steam. Then we'd be in a good place and attract people in a good place.'

It's easy to blame societal influences and bad parents for making us clingy but that's only part of the cause. There is one school of thought that we are all prone to getting hooked on an unavailable person or a relationship. It comes from the renowned psychiatrist Harville Hendrix. He believes we all harbour an image of our ideal partner in our subconscious and calls this fantasy person our 'imago'. He or she represents snapshots of significant people in our lives and our childhood caregivers. His Imago theory predicts that we unconsciously select a partner with the same positive and negative traits of our primary childhood caregivers because we are trying to satisfy the emotional needs not fulfilled in childhood. If our parents were emotionally or physically unavailable, often we go for unavailable men or women.

Hendrix predicts that we live life continually looking for our imago. We believe there is someone out there who can solve all our problems and love us unconditionally, even if we don't wash. If we don't learn to manage this, we walk around in a constant state of longing. But if we do meet someone who represents our imago – unless we have the strongest addiction-proof brain – we're doomed. So we're damned if we find our imago and damned if we don't. Basically, we're a race of love addicts.

CHAPTER 16

Love Inc.

You know when you see a picture of a hammock on a paradise holiday island brochure? Maybe you don't make a habit of looking in upmarket brochures. Just any old picture of a hammock will do. There it is, swaying in the breeze beside the turquoise blue sea, waves lapping. We're led to believe that sitting in one takes you to the most peaceful, happy, carefree, cocktail-tainted resting place. But if you've ever lounged in one of those mouldy string nets, you'll know they take 20 minutes to get into, there's mosquito eggs in the gaps, and if you ever get into a remotely tolerable position you can't reach your drink or your sunglasses.

I think marriage has been sold to us in much the same way. Somehow, someone or something has projected images of long-term, cohabiting, lifelong partnerships – ideally with a few well-behaved children in tow – as the route to a happy, successful and respectable life. Great if you want that. Not so great if either you don't want it, or haven't even thought about it. For some people the thing that's supposed to puff your heart out is actually the cause of frustration and anguish.

So, how has this prescription for happiness emerged? It's a result of anachronistic historical values more suited to a different era, our human susceptibility to the foibles of romantic love and a judgemental social climate, which refuses to accept that anyone else's desires and characters can be different to its own. I call this big cumulative force Love Inc. It's like a corporate superpower that manufactures and commercialises ideas for romantic and sexual satisfaction. The more people buy into its products, the larger and more influential it becomes.

Love Inc.'s bestseller is the Hollywood love story, in which single people always get together with their Prince/Princess. Estranged couples always get back together and anyone who has an affair either redeems himself or gets killed. Hollywood movies, chick-lit romance and even the celebrity gossip in newspapers and magazines are all remakes of the fairytale staple where a Princess meets her Prince and both live happily ever after. The credits roll and the book always ends with an embrace. We are left believing the rest of their lives will be lived happily ever after, but that's just like a session break in the grander story of love.

Fairytale love stories are deliciously appealing to our romantic natures and endless quest for happiness but they don't give us a real understanding of love and relationships in the modern world. Love Inc.'s marketing ignores the science – that when you're so enamored with someone that you really think you're going to feel like this forever, in fact your brain is behaving in the same way as a crack addict. It ignores the historical facts that long-term partnerships had nothing to do with love throughout most of human history bar the last 200 years and also the strengthening wave of resistance. Fewer people are choosing marriage or even full-time relationships. Even those in relationships are doing so in new ways to suit them – they're experimenting with open marriage, living apart because they can, defining their dynamic with a monthly allowance or creating D/s contracts!

Love Inc. bombards us with pictures of smiling couples in shampoo adverts and holiday brochures. We open a newspaper and see images of celebrity couples hand in hand, accompanied by gossip on who is dating whom as if love is the most important thing in their lives. What about other things such as friends, homes, holidays, aspirations? We are led to believe that a relationship is the most important thing to aspire to.

Fifty-year anniversaries are celebrated with great acclaim even though the individuals may hate each other. Love Inc. leads us to believe that if a relationship doesn't last until death does us part, we have in some way failed despite scientific, historical and sociological evidence to prove long-lasting love is rare.

Should longevity be the only parameter on which to base the success of a relationship? For me, what constitutes a fulfilling relationship is how we appreciate and respect each other, what we can teach each other and the experiences and conversations we share. Longevity may matter for those bringing up children but if you think about it, our child-raising years are a small part of our romantic lifespan. There's no need to instill the strict policies of Love Inc. into teenagers and 20-somethings – after all, a third of them are going to live beyond 100. Similarly, once children have left home, their middle-aged parents will increasingly find themselves on the dating scene again. Through death or divorce, the 50+ demographic is the largest growing sector of Internet daters.

Love Inc. also creates brands. We have 'The One', 'Mr Right', 'My Other Half', 'Someone to Grow Old With', 'My Rock'. A relationship has been made into a must-have accessory. We feel inadequate if we don't have the prototype of perfection; we suffer couple envy. We obsess over celebrity love lives. How do *they* do it? We pore over relationship self-help books; we read tips on how to inject passion back into our relationship.

Love Inc. also tells us that our parents did it better. Our grandparents didn't get divorced, don't you know? Today we are a 'fragmented society' and it's all the fault of those disconnected people who keep casting off Love Inc.'s products and trying more bespoke versions. Marriage is apparently 'in crisis'. Crisis, what crisis? Some of the so-called victims of our 'epidemic of loneliness' are actually glad they live alone! Single parents in the 'divorce casualties' have admitted their lives were turned around when they found the courage to break free.

Michael Cobb, the long-term singleton who wrote *Single: Arguments of the Uncoupled*, goes so far to say our must-marry mantra is a result of totalitarianism: 'It's about coercion and control. If you can get people anxious and persuade them all to have the same fears and desires, you can market a way of living.'

And market we do. The dating industry was estimated to be worth £105 million a year in the UK in 2011, according to the market research giant Mintel. Bookshelves overspill with relationship self-help volumes. Every newspaper has a sex and relationships agony aunt. Live TV shows attract millions of viewers for hooking people up. Once *Blind Date*, now it's *Take Me Out*.

Relationship advice books follow two themes – 'How to find Mr Right' and 'How to Make it Last'. Oh no, there's a third! The ones that market themselves to single men and women, instructing them on 'how to enjoy a single life' – as if we need a lesson on how to live in the default state in which we were born!

No one advises us to adopt an individual approach to relationships; no one gives leeway to those who may not aspire to sharing a home, those for whom monogamy isn't important or those who feel that a relationship could be number two in their lives. But the big monster machine that is Love Inc. tells us that our relationships must come first. It reminds me of the John Grisham novel *The Firm*, where everything about employees' lives had to pale into insignificance once they signed up.

When I've had boyfriends, serious ones, not just lovers, I have loved them dearly but I haven't unquestionably put them first. Sometimes I have. But there are also times when I put my career first. Or friends first. Or training for a triathlon. Perhaps one day I'll become a Greenpeace activist and I'll put that first. Maybe one day I'll need to care for a family member and I'll put them first.

You may ask, might a relationship wilt through lack of attention? But I'd prefer that to one which became all-consuming. Two of the interviewees in Eric Klineberg's book *Going Solo* stand out for me because they faced such a predicament. Both had met someone they cared for deeply after being alone for a long time but they were equally concerned that taking things further with their new love interests would have consequences for their autonomy.

In both cases, it wasn't as if they doubted the person they had met, it was that they didn't want to go past a point where moving in would be expected of them. Eventually they had to choose whether to succumb to their partner's demands to move in or end the relationship totally. Both chose the latter because their autonomy was too valuable. I found it sad that this manufactured ideal of what love should be is so prototypical that it drove them away.

I am no longer in a relationship with the 'serious boyfriend' whom I met while writing this book. But that does not mean that I feel 'it didn't work out'. The experience was enriching and enjoyable and I savour the memory of integrating my life for a short time with a wonderful person but I also know that it wasn't what I wanted forever. I didn't consider the end of the relationship a failure. Sad, yes, but success of a relationship should not just be judged on longevity alone.

One of the big things I found myself benefiting from after starting a 'proper relationship' was the social approval. Family were very chuffed indeed that I was at last 'with someone' and not writing any more memoirs about my sex life. People at parties seem relieved when I said 'I have a boyfriend'. As one half of a couple, I was less of a threat and less of an enigma. My sports masseuse was happy, naturally. And the comments about ageing with felines totally ceased!

There were lots of other positive things about being in a relationship. But deep down there was always the wild, mammalian me that longed to release myself back into the wild, uncultivated world of singledom. I missed the nomadic feeling of being untethered to anyone or anything.

As one (happily) married friend said to me, 'The thing I miss about being single is the thought that you can go out one evening and it's possible to flatline into a completely different life.' I don't think my friend actually wanted to do so but she liked the fantasy that she could; that she could have her fairytale moment again. You see the most exciting thing about the fairytale is the part where the Prince and Princess get together. Once they've kissed, the story becomes so dull that it ends.

Like everyone, I too am tempted by Love Inc's blurb. I too think it would be wonderful to meet a soulmate who sychronises with my life on every level. But as William the bachelor said in Chapter One, the reality is always different. I'll let u into a secret. I always cry at weddings because it hits home that I haven't got what those people have. I haven't found my fairytale ending and I'm not nuzzling someone special for the first dance on the dancefloor, tripping over my white wedding gown while everyone says 'ahhhh'. Like Julie, the glamorous single mother who never married, whom we met in Chapter One, a part of me is sad that I don't think I'll ever have that. But there is also relief that I won't. If I had to choose between having love but feeling like my wings were clipped or craving love a little but being free, I'd choose the latter without hesitation.

I sometimes worry that like the romance addicts we met in the previous chapter, I too am addicted to the honeymoon highs of new love. That I am a dopamine chaser, all to ready to replace solid, reliable boyfriends with shiny and new lovers. I usually get to around 18 months of coupledom and then I have the thirst to play the game of new love again. I'm well aware it's a gamble. It's total exhilaration if it goes well. It's utterly soul destroying if a new love interest doesn't text.

I used to chastise myself for getting bored so quickly. Why couldn't I be content with settling with a wonderful man who loves me, building a home and riding out the good times and bad together? But now I think my formula for shorter but equally generous love affairs is the one that suits our natures better. The evidence I have visited throughout this book certainly points at this as a better model. Scientifically we know that new love is powerful, addictive, frenzied and euphoric but it doesn't last. Historically we know that long-term partnership has never been about love and compatibility. Socially, we know that less people are choosing conventional coupledom and are carving their own paths of romantic fulfilment. There are a number of pioneers testing new formulas for a relationship designed to prevent becoming swallowed up by it. The likes of LAT couples like Olivia and Alan, who love each other but readily admit that they do not put being together above other things in their lives. Or Tuppy and Anthony, who hope to remain together for their winter years but allow each other the pleasure to pursue lovers. Or the sperm donor mothers who consider a relationship something they will find later once the more important business of raising a child has been ticked.

The difficulty that love pioneers like us face is that most couples have bearings that bind them together – a shared address, kids, a shared surname. Each additional responsibility is another building block that makes it harder for them to crumble. Because I don't want all those things, my relationships become ethereal. There is nothing to hold them together other than love and trust. I wonder if we stack these building blocks because it settles our own insecurities? As one man put it during one of the many and varied interviews for this book: 'No man will tell you this, but if a man asks for marriage it's because it's the most secure way of holding onto her.'

LOVE INC.

I hate to sound unromantic, but whether we choose to stay in a relationship or not is just an equation: what nourishment we get from it versus what we give up. I liked being in love very much but not enough to give up the freedom and opportunism of being single. For others – probably the majority – it's a price worth paying.

If I wanted children, I'd have found someone to have them with by now. If I was the sort of person who wasn't good on my own or, like Cate the submissive we met earlier, if I needed someone to boot me out of bed every day to get going because I couldn't do it myself, I'd be living with someone right now. If I lived in a village where everyone around me got married, I'd probably follow suit. Maybe if I hadn't had a career redirection to journalism and I was still drumming my fingers at an accountant's desk in a steady routine, I'd bore easily and I'd want to see my boyfriend more. If I lived 100 years ago and I couldn't earn as much as a man, take out a loan, vote, get access to contraception, travel or live alone, too right I'd get married!

Love Inc. generates a one-size-fits-all model of relationship but we can all do better than that. We heard how asexuals felt something was wrong with them for not wanting the sort of sexual relationships their friends had. Also how bachelors like William and the 'hemmed-in' philanderer Mike found the reality of marriage oppressive. We heard from divorcées who admitted they had only married because they felt that's what they should do, and it made them miserable. And we heard from polyamorous and open couples who felt stigmatised when they told colleagues they could love more than one person.

We are the first generation to be able to truly enjoy the opportunity to live relationships in different ways. Perhaps in the future the socio-economic climate, over-population, energy shortages or other horrors will once more render full-time, cohabiting, socially binding partnerships necessary again. But they're not here yet and so I'm going to organise my love affairs according to the demands of real modern life.

Love Inc. will keep on trading, flogging us books on outdated and ill-founded formulae for achieving happiness through a fulfilling life-long relationship. Commentators will still deride anyone who doesn't aspire to the exemplar of everlasting love with a shared front door. We'll continue to sleepwalk into marriage and kids without questioning alternatives. But I will continue to be a relationship revolutionary because I know that as much as I'd like to believe in the fairytale, as much as I like the idea that there is one being who will be my life inspiration and provide all the answers, the more I delve into the mysterious matter of love, the more I realise that person is me.

Further Reading

BOOKS

A Strange Stirring: The Feminine Mystique and American Women at the Dawn of the 1960s, Stephanie Coontz (Basic Books, 2011).

Anxiety Attacks: Conquering Your Insecurities, Dr Lucy Atcheson (Hay House UK, July 2009).

Atlas of World Cultures, George Peter Murdoch (University of Pittsburgh Press, May 1981).

Bachelor Girl: 100 Years of Breaking the Rules – A Social History of Living Single, Betsy Israel (Perennial/HarperCollins, 2003).

Bachelors: The Psychology of Men Who Haven't Married, Charles A. Waehler (Greenwood Press, October 1996).

BDSM: The Naked Truth, Dr Charley Ferrer (Institute of Pleasure, July 2011).

Celebrating the Family: Ethnicity, Consumer Culture, and Family Rituals, Elizabeth H. Pleck (Harvard University Press, July 2000).

Committed: A Sceptic Makes Peace With Marriage, Elizabeth Gilbert (Bloomsbury Publishing, January 2010).

Dangerous Women: The Guide to Modern Life, Claire Convil and Liz Hoggord (Orion Publishing, 2011).

Ever Dated a Psycho? Paul Duddridge (Short Books, February 2008).

Fear of Flying, Erica Jong (Vintage, new edition, June 1994).

Fear of Freedom, Eriic Fromm (Routledge Classics, May 2001).

Female Chauvinist Pigs: Women and the Rise of Raunch Culture, Ariel Levy (Pocket Books, June 2006).

Francis Bacon: The Major Works, edited by Brian Vickers (OUP Oxford, May 2008).

Going Solo: The Extraordinary Rise and Surprising Appeal of Living Alone, Eric Klinenberg (Penguin Press, April 2012).

Honey Money: The Power of Erotic Capital, Catherine Hakim (Allen Lane, August 2011).

How To Think More About Sex, Alain de Botton (Macmillan, May 2012).

I Can Barely Take Care of Myself: Tales From a Happy Life Without Kids, Jen Kirkman. (Simon & Schuster, April 2013).

I'd Rather be Single than Settle: Satisfied Solitude and How to Achieve It., Emily Dubberley (Fusion Press, 2006).

Is It Love or Is It Addiction? The Book That Changed the Way We Think About Romance and Intimacy, Brenda Schaeffer (Hazelden Publishing & Educational Services, 3rd edition, May 2009).

Living Dolls: The Return of Sexism, Natasha Walters (Virago, May 2011).

Love and Limerence: The Experience of Being in Love, Dorothy Tennov (Scarborough House; 2nd edition, December 1998).

Love Junkie: A Memoir, Rachel Resnick (Bloomsbury, November 2008).

Marriage, a History: How Love Conquered Marriage, Stephanie Coontz (Penguin, February 2006).

Marriage Confidential: The Post-Romantic Age of Workhorse Wives, Royal Children, Undersexed Spouses, and Rebel Couples Who Are Rewriting the Rules, Pamela Susan Haag (HarperCollins, May 2011).

Men Who Can't Love: How to Recognize a Commitment-phobic Man before He Breaks Your Heart, Julia Sokol and Steven Carter (M. Evans & Co Inc, new edition, November 2003).

Mistresses: A History of the Other Woman, Elizabeth Abbott (Overlook Hardcover, September 2011).

Mother Nature: Maternal Instincts and How They Affect the Human Species, Sarah Blaffer Hrdy (Ballantine Books, September 2000).

New Rules: Searching for Self-fulfilment in a World Turned Upside Down, Daniel Yankelovich (Bantam Books, 1982).

No More Silly Love Songs: A Realist's Guide to Romance, Anouchka Grose (Portobello Books, January 2011).

Paper Houses: A Memoir of the 70s and Beyond, Michele Roberts (Virago Press Ltd., July 2008).

Plato's Symposium: A New Translation, Robin Waterfield (Oxford World's Classics, January 2009).

Quirkyalone: A Manifesto of Uncompromising Romantics, Sasha Cagen. (Harper One, January 2006).

Rewriting the Rules: An Integrative Guide to Love, Sex and Relationships, Meg Barker (Routledge, August 2012).

Sex and Love Addicts Anonymous: The Basic Text for the Augustine Fellowship, The Augustine Fellowship (Augustine Fellowship, June 1986).

Sex at Dawn: How We Mate, Why We Stray and What It Means for Modern Relationships, Christopher Ryan and Cacilda Jethá (HarperCollins, February 2011).

Single: Arguments for the Uncoupled, Michael Cobb (NYU Press, September 2012).

Singled Out: How Singles Are Stereotyped, Stigmatized, and Ignored, and Still Live Happily Ever After, Bella Depaulo (St. Martin's Press, November 2006).

Sinners? Scroungers? Saints? Unmarried Motherhood in Twentieth-Century England, Patricia Thane and Tanya Evans (OUP Oxford, May 2012).

Sugar Daddy Diaries: When a Fantasy Became an Obsession, Helen Croydon (Mainstream Publishing, March 2011).

The Best-Kept Secret: Men and Women's Stories of Lasting Love, Professor Janet Reibstein (Bloomsbury Publishing PLC, February 2006).

The Changing Lives of American Women, Steven D. McLaughlin et al. (University of North Carolina Press, 1988) (USA).

The End of Men: And the Rise of Women, Hannah Rosin (Viking, October 2012).

The Ethical Slut: Guide to Infinite Sexual Possibilities, Dossie Easton (Greenery Press, December 1997).

The Evolution of Desire: Strategies of Human Mating, David M. Buss (Basic Books, January 1995).

The Fear of Freedom, Erich Fromm (Routledge Classics, May 2001).

The Female Brain, Louanne Brizendine (Bantam, January 2008).

The Golden Bough: A Study in Magic and Religion, Sir James Frazer (Oxford World's Classics, February 2009).

The Lifestyle: A Look at the Erotic Rites of Swingers, Terry Gould (Vintage Canada, 1999).

The Marriage Crisis, Ernest Groves (Longmans, Green & Co. , January, 1928) (USA).

The Marriage Delusion: The Fraud of the Rings, Mike Buchanan (LPS Publishing 2009).

The New Rules: Internet, Playfairs and Erotic Power, Catherine Hakim (Gibson Square, 2012).

The Paradox of Love, Pascal Bruckner (Princeton University Press, February 2012).

The Seducer's Diary, Soren Kierkegaard (Penguin Classics, August 2007).

The Sex Contract: The Evolution of Human Behavior, Helen E. Fisher (William Morrow & Co., reprint edition, January 1983).

The Spectacle of Nature: Landscape and Bourgeois Culture in Nineteenth-century France, Nicholas Green (Manchester University Press, July 1990.

The Whole Woman, Germaine Greer (Black Swan, February 2007).

Turned On, Lucy Dent (Doubleday, March 2013).

Understanding Asexuality, Anthony F. Bogaert (Rowman & Littlefield Publishers, August 2012).

Well-being: Productivity and Happiness at Work, Ivan Robertson and Professor Cary Cooper (Palgrave Macmillan, April 2011).

What Makes Women Happy, Fay Weldon (Harper Perennial, January 2008

Why Have Kids?: A New Mom Explores the Truth About

Parenting and Happiness, Jessica Valenti (New Harvest, September 2012).

Why Him? Why Her? How to Find and Keep Lasting Love, Helen Fisher. (Oneworld Publications, February 2011).

Why You're Not Married Yet: The Straight Talk You Need to Get the Relationship You Deserve, Tracy McMillan (Ballantine Books, March 2013).

Women Who Love Too Much, Robin Norwood (Arrow, September 2004)

SURVEYS, REPORTS AND ARTICLES

'Articles from the Journal: Stories With a Withdrawal Focus', The Augustine Fellowship, Sex and Love Addicts Anonymous. 2004

'Childlessness in Europe', Catherine Hakim (report for The Economic and Social Research Council).

'General Lifestyle Survey', 2011 (released March 2013), Office for National Statistics.

'Lovegeist Love Landscape: A Study of Contemporary Dating in Modern Britain', Match.com. 2009

The Polyamory Project, Jemima Wilcox (self-published). June 2012

'The Singleton Society: Targeting the Bridget Jones Generation', Clare Staunton, Future Foundation, May 2008.

'Who Will Love Me When I'm 64?' Relate and New Philanthropy Capital. June 2013